Community Nursing and Health Care

INSIGHTS AND INNOVATIONS

D0147680

Edited by
Val Hyde

Institute of Health Sciences
University of Plymouth, UK

A member of the Hodder Headline Group
LONDON

First published in Great Britain in 2001 by
Arnold, a member of the Hodder Headline Group,
338 Euston Road, London NW1 3BH

http://www.arnoldpublishers.com

© 2001 Arnold

British Library Cataloguing in Publication Data
A catalogue record for this book is available from the British Library

ISBN 0 340 76011 7 (pb)

1 2 3 4 5 6 7 8 9 10

Commissioning Editor: Aileen Parlane
Production Editor: Rada Radojicic
Production Controller: Martin Kerans
Cover Design: Terry Griffiths

Typeset in Palatino by J&L Composition Ltd, Filey, North Yorkshire
Printed and bound in Great Britain by MPG Books Ltd, Bodmin, Cornwall

What do you think about this book? Or any other Arnold title?
Please send your comments to feedback.arnold@hodder.co.uk

Contents

Contributors

Marc A. Cornock
Principal Lecturer
Institute of Health Studies
University of Plymouth
England

Clare Cotter
Practising District Nurse
South Devon Healthcare Trust
England

Kath Hutchinson
Health Visitor
Reading
England

Val Hyde
Principal Lecturer
Institute of Health Studies
University of Plymouth
England

Kate Lock
Primary Care Development Manager
East Devon Primary Care Trust
England

Lorly McClure
Lecturer in Health and Social Care
University of Reading
England

Carolyn Mason
Nursing Officer – Public Health
Northern Ireland Department of Health, Social Services and Public Safety
Northern Ireland

Paul Parkin
Senior Lecturer
Department of Health Studies
Brunel University
England

David Pontin
Senior Lecturer
Institute of Health Studies
University of the West of England
Bristol
England

Paul Swift
Research Fellow – Learning Disabilities
Institute for Applied Health and Social Policy
Kings College
London
England

Sandy Tinson
Director of Clinical Development
Reading Primary Care Trust
Reading
England

Rosie Walsh
Nurse Facilitator
Cornwall and Isles of Scilly Health Authority
England

Mary Watkins
Head of Institute of Health Studies
University of Plymouth
England

Diana White
Practising District Nurse
Exeter NHS Community Trust
England

Val Woodward
Senior Lecturer, Community Nursing
Institute of Health Studies
University of Plymouth
England

Introduction

This book seeks to capture the key issues and trends for community nurses within the most dynamic context since the inception of the NHS. It is written by a variety of professionals, each contributing through their professional roles to the development of contemporary community nursing. Timely insights are offered into the challenge to 'redesign services around the needs of the patient' (DOH, 1999).

This 'redesigning' process requires more than a new approach; it requires a significant cultural change to create enabling organisations which can deliver the agenda. The first four chapters consider current health policy and examine the ways in which it contributes to or detracts from the creation of such organisations. The following three chapters then explore new opportunities for partnership working, and the next three particular challenges for today's and tomorrow's community nurses. The last chapter, written at the publication of The NHS Plan, then considers the future of community nursing and some of the new issues that pose fresh challenges to the practice of community health care nursing.

In the opening chapter, Kate Lock and Diana White provide an overview of key current developments, enabling the reader to understand these within the evolving political context. Several possible areas of expansion for nurses are examined and new opporunities for nurses are highlighted. It is concluded however, that the measure of their success will be determined largely by the adaptability of nurses.

In the next chapter, Carolyn Mason addresses one of the government's main emphases: public health. It is argued that public health encompasses a range of activities including health protection, prevention, health education, healthy public policy and community empowerment. After a thorough analysis of relevant factors, it is noted that community nursing in the UK appears to be primarily client and family centred, rather than population centred. Readers are given substantive guidance as to how they might increase their capacity to meet the public health agenda.

A model of a population centred approach is offered by Sandy Tinson in the next chapter, in her examination of a new agenda for action in relation to health needs assessment. Some illuminating discussion clarifies this problematic concept and a number of different perspectives are contrasted (e.g. those of sociologists, economists and epidemiologists). Helpful examples from practice and a valuable case study illustrate the impact that can be brought to bear through effective health needs assessment, on the health and life chances of those living in the community.

In Chapter 4, Mary Watkins considers the challenges that are presented to healthcare professionals who provide community care to individuals with mental health problems. Problems and weaknesess of past service provision are drawn upon to consider ways in which the NHS framework for mental health and the primary care standards might be turned into reality. Case studies from everyday practice highlight the benefits and appropriateness of collaborative working.

In the first of three chapters focusing on partnership working, Lorly McClure acknowledges family caregivers as co-experts in care. The chapter majors on the caregiving experience from the family caregiver's perspective and a stimulating debate is presented which questions the extent to which a partnership between community nurses and carers is possible. Lorly encourages readers to enhance their practice by learning from the caring ethos that is securely rooted in the enduring care that takes place within family relationships.

David Swift and David Pontin's chapter is embedded in the practical experiences of community nurses working as care managers in Somerset. Some helpful case studies are used to illustrate the ethical issues that nurse assessors face. The chapter seeks to redress the lack of research into the far reaching effects of the NHS and Community Care Act 1990 for both clients and care workers. A number of models of care management are appraised and key outcomes of specific projects are identified.

The next chapter by Paul Parkin outlines the position of the community nurse in the patient's home, who is subjected to formal and informal forces. Informal, social relations systems located in the home are seen to generate a genuine need for reciprocity to retrieve status balance within a potentially unequal relationship. Paul argues cogently that since the planning of healthcare should always be on the basis of need, the giving and receiving of gifts should be allowed as an important aspect of all social relations.

Rosie Walsh acknowledges that the current climate of innovation and development in primary care has been encouraged by the government which has emphasised in particular nurse led services. Her chapter is a timely exploration of the complex concept of autonomous practice which, consequent to the development of extended/expanded nurse roles in the community, gives rise to much debate. Accountability and autonomy are discussed in relation to various issues including clinical governance, codes of conduct, legal issues, and professional changes.

This theme is continued in the next chapter by Marc Cornock whose explanation of the working of legal and ethical systems clarifies the framework in which community nurses practice. Marc emphasises that the purpose of ethics and law in relation to healthcare is the protection of patient's rights as well as the rights of the nurse. Many of the recurring problematic areas such as confidentiality, informed consent, and receiving of gifts are expounded in this chapter, with the help of examples from practice.

In the next chapter Val Woodward notes that the community is an environment that is increasingly influenced by governmental policies seeking efficiency and effectiveness; the evidence-based movement is therefore highlighted as the way forward for all healthcare professionals. The chapter gives an overview of the nature of evidence, the concept of evidence-based practice, the clinical governance initiative, and the relevance of these to community practitioners. In addition to containing a wealth of comprehensive and current knowledge, the chapter constitutes an excellent practical guide to community professionals who wish to develop their practice for the benefit of their clients.

In the final chapter Val Hyde and Clare Cotter consider the recently published NHS Plan, and discuss some of the key factors that may influence the extent to which community nurses respond to the challenges presented. They conclude that the biggest challenge to the success of the NHS Plan is the breaking down of barriers. Without real and continued commitment to collaborative working, Val and Clare warn that none of the five challenges addressed by the plan can be fully met.

A strength of the book is its revisitation of key themes from different perspectives, for example clinical governance is included in Chapters 1, 8 and 10 which complement each other and assist the reader to grasp the whole picture. A further example is the giving and receiving of gifts which is set in a legal context by Marc Cornock in Chapter 7, and a social context by Paul Parkin in Chapter 9. The book adds to the body of current literature on community nursing, offering insights into the key issues within the relationship between community healthcare nurses, their clients and their carers, and the changing relationships that they must build with other professionals to enable community care to be 'redesigned around the patient'.

Community nursing in the new NHS

1

Kate Lock and Diana White

Introduction

The last two years have seen a rapid change in the community health care services in the UK. The Blair Labour government promised a radical change in the way that health services out of hospital would be delivered. The following year saw such a flurry of policy changes, central health service guidelines (albeit usually two months late) and structural change that it was hard to believe the rhetoric about 'evolution not revolution'. This 'policy-itis' may have subsided a little, and it is time to take stock of what has been achieved and how this might affect community nursing in the first years of the next millennium.

Great things are forecast for community nursing: an expanded public health role, greater involvement in strategic decision-making, the forging of partnerships with agencies we were so recently embattled against and an increasing need to be self-critical about the quality and responsiveness of our work. Community nursing will be judged on its ability to meet the challenge of the changes and the impact of these on our clients.

ORIGINS OF CHANGE

Despite the shifts, there is far more continuity in the changes in the NHS than new Labour would lead us to believe. In 1990, the then Conservative government passed legislation to bring in Trust status for hospitals and community services, and GP fundholding in primary care – the purchaser/provider split in the NHS. The same bill (NHS and Community Care Act 1990) required Social Services to divide similarly, although the implementation of this was delayed until 1993. The impact of these changes was enormous.

First, it clearly defined those shaping the future of health services – the health authorities – and gave them independence from those who were involved with the daily running of operations. Once health authorities were then merged with Family Health Service authorities (mid-1980s), whole health service planning was made possible. However, the strictures of GP fundholding and the competitive atmosphere of the NHS made real change in the direction of services very difficult to achieve.

Second, trust status, whilst it bred competitiveness which was intensely frustrating to practitioners, did for the first time enable some community services to grow an identity of their own, unhindered by their hospital neigh-bours. Community trusts, many of which had mental health services and learning disability services within their remit, experimented with models of service delivery not previously possible. In some places fundholding proved a brake to this process, stopping the flexible usage of staff. In others, though, it proved a stimulus for change. Since trusts were no longer obliged to oper-ate to a national framework, flexible management systems were possible. Self-managed teams of community nurses were allowed to develop and nurses were able to develop new clinical skills and use them in creative new ways in conjunction with their colleagues in general practice.

Fundholding practices often saw the benefit of directly employing more nurses, and the growth of practice nurses that had preceded the 1990 Act con-tinued apace. For the most part, these were nurses without community nurs-ing qualifications. In response to the health promotion targets, many GPs allowed practice nurses to take on substantial responsibilities in the manage-ment of patients with chronic disease (asthma and diabetes, for example) and expand their role in health promotion (well-men and well-women clinics, smoking cessation clinics). GP practices were paid on activity – outcomes of care were seldom monitored beyond practice audit. Evidence now shows that health promotion activity spawned under this system tended to target those from the middle classes who were healthier, leaving untouched those in greatest need of these services.

Implementation of the 1990 Community Care Act also forged changes to community nursing. It brought two conflicting pressures to bear. The move to care management and the imperative to assess and manage all clients, opened the possibilities for health professionals to co-operate fully with social ser-vices. This led to the formation of close alliances of health and social services colleagues in community mental health teams and teams for those working with learning-disabled clients. However, the Act also pushed a wedge between social and health care by insisting on very different budget and ser-vice streams, so that in some areas it became essential to categorize every activity as either health or social care. This led to some madness – 'Is this a health or social bath?', 'A health or social commode?' – which made life for district nurses, in particular, very difficult. However, other areas of the Act brought a rigor to planning in the health service, and the role of rehabilitation in enabling older people to return to full activity was now emphasized, as opposed to the caring but containing attitude which had characterized many day hospital facilities previously.

In conclusion, the 1980s were a time of change for community health ser-vices, for although the changes brought the necessity of increasing partner-ship between agencies more clearly to mind, structures were built in that made it difficult. Structures were created to loosen central control of services but these also put in place obstacles to that control. For practitioners work-ing during this time, however, it demonstrated the necessity for them to embrace change – albeit critically – so that the new structures might better meet the needs of the local population, although the results did not always meet expectations.

NEW LABOUR – *OUR HEALTHIER NATION/SAVING LIVES*

The new government did not come to power unprepared. The Blairite shadow cabinet had worked with the sure expectation of winning the election. As the Department of Education had systems set up in the spring to accommodate David Blunkett and his dog, so Frank Dobson's Department of Health team had fully formed plans as they moved into the Department of Health on 3 May 1997. Policies descended thick and fast. By February 1998 we had the broad outline and substantial detail of the changes planned. Importantly, the changes in education, social services and local government were also known and there were common themes that threaded through all documents. All agencies were charged with a statutory duty of partnership and a requirement to target services at those socially excluded, with an implicit or explicit admission that previously services had been best-suited to those who needed them least. Action zones in health, education and employment were to be formed to focus the minds on those in areas of greatest disadvantage. The documents all called for increased public consultation and for greater responsiveness of services to the varied needs of the community.

The fact that the thinking was 'joined-up' made the changes far more likely to be carried through. Whether that will mean that the government will reach its objective has yet to be seen.

Parallel to these changes were the moves toward devolution of power to Scotland, Wales and Northern Ireland. This chapter will concentrate on changes in England, but Scotland and Wales are having similar, but not identical changes made to their systems. Of course, Scotland had a different system of health care structures under previous administrations, whereas Wales had previously been similar to England. Since the stalling of the Northern Ireland Assembly, no changes have been instituted in Northern Ireland, but these will no doubt follow, when and if the power-sharing agreements hold long enough for business to commence.

In England the building block of the changes in health is the White Paper, *Saving Lives* (DOH, 1999a), previously the longest running Green paper, *Our Healthier Nation* (DOH, 1998b). This replaced the Conservative *Health of the Nation* (1992), which described targets for health promotion. *Health of the Nation* (DOH, 1992) was a document centred on the effect individuals could have on their health, and the way the NHS should support this change. *Saving Lives* (DOH, 1999a) takes the brave step of acknowledging that individual choice, although central to the debate, is only one element in explaining the health of the public. It sets out community and national responsibilities needed to improve health, with the theme of concentrating on partnership working and targeting those in most need. Although it requires the NHS to act on four target areas (mental health – reduce suicide, accidents – reduce childhood attendance for accidents at health facilities, cardiovascular disease – cut the death rates for stroke and heart attack, cancer – cut the death rates for specific cancers), it boldly admits that these targets are not particularly ambitious. However, the radical change it calls for is the concentration on upstream thinking. A colleague describes this as 'not waiting until someone falls into the river to fish them out, but stopping them falling in'.

The Acheson Report (DOH, 1997a) gave the essential evidence-based foundation for this upstream thinking, making clear the links between ill health and poverty. *Saving Lives* (DOH, 1999a) looks at schemes to increase smoking cessation, in particular among the poorest, increasing the availability of low-cost high-quality food, walk to school initiatives, availability of contraception and sexual health education for teenagers – aimed, again, at those in greatest need, the poorest in the community. It also challenges the NHS to work in partnership with all other agencies, to consult more widely with the public on the right shape of services and to use the expertise of patients to inform and support others (the 'expert patient'; DOH, 1999a).

Crucially for community nursing, *Saving Lives* (DOH, 1999a) sees a central role for health visitors and school nurses in taking up this public health work. It expects them to be at the forefront of change in community health, working with colleagues from social services, education, local authorities and the voluntary sector to build healthy communities. From the time in the mid-1980s when 'society' was declared dead by Margaret Thatcher, we have now a government which describes a role for health professionals in creating a healthy society.

Some were disappointed to see only health visiting and school nursing described so explicitly. Many district nurses, community mental health nurses and practice nurses – to name but three – saw themselves as change agents in the community. It remains to be seen if even health visitors and school nurses will be allowed the latitude to work as public health workers by managers used to productivity targets on face-to-face contacts.

Making a Difference (DOH, 1999b) clarified the process of this change. The paper also required the NHS to assess local health needs in far more thorough ways than previously. In some places, health visitors had always assessed need, creating community profiles, but health needs assessment by the public health departments of health authorities had previously been confined to assessing the impact of health interventions rather than the health of public. The explanations of so-called 'variations in health' were not encouraged, nor were the effects of poverty or deprivation acknowledged as important in the delivery of health services. *Saving Lives* (DOH, 1999a), with other initiatives, sought to reverse this tendency, emphasizing the need to assess the health of the public, to explore the effects of poverty and social exclusion on health and to work with other agencies to deliver this assessment in a way that all agencies could have an active role. It had been hoped that needs assessment would be able to describe local issues. However, in the welter of national and district priorities, it has become increasingly clear that scope for local action has been severely curtailed. This might mean more careful local planning to fit in with district objectives, or it may result in yet another form of imposed decision-making on communities. The role of community nursing in health needs assessment is explained more fully in Chapter 3.

WHITE PAPER/HEALTH ACT 1999

The mechanism by which the new Labour government envisaged these changes was laid out in the White Paper, *The New NHS – Modern and Dependable*

(DOH, 1997b), paradoxically, published in December 1997. The speed of the release of this White Paper, less than nine months after the election, displayed no lack of mature thinking on health service structures. Much detail then followed in health service circulars over the next 18 months, with the Health Act becoming law at the end of the summer session of 1999.

HEALTH IMPROVEMENT PROGRAMMES

The White Paper redraws the structural map of the NHS. Health authorities are charged with drawing up priorities for their areas. To do this they must work with all other agencies (health Trusts, social services, local authorities, the police, the voluntary sector etc.) and the public to produce a plan for health improvement for their district. The first health improvement programmes (HImPs) were published in March 1999. They varied from short booklets to huge tomes. Some dealt exclusively with the *Our Healthier Nation* (DOH, 1998b) health improvement strategy; others concentrated on defining service structure and targets for service delivery. Most worked in the middle ground between. All had the requisite players signed up to priorities – a real achievement given the very tight timescales.

PRIMARY CARE GROUP (PCG) TO PRIMARY CARE TRUST (PCT) STATUS

The White Paper describes the formation of primary care groups (PCGs), run by boards of general practitioners, nurses and social services managers who act as commissioners of health services – both primary and secondary. This clearly puts community health practitioners in positions of power in forming a 'primary care-led NHS'. It asks practitioners also to take a corporate view of health improvement – to balance financial resources and improve quality.

HImPs define the priorities within which the PCGs must work. A PCG can operate at one of four levels; in effect, however, only three will exist. The vast majority of the 481 PCGs in England started at Level 2 in April 1999 – taking responsibility for between 40% and 60% of the commissioning budget, but remaining subcommittees of the Health Authority. April 2000 saw 17 PCGs move to Level 4 and become PCTs – legally freestanding bodies which are responsible for their entire budget and are able to operate as providers as well as commissioners of services. It seems that most PCTs will initially only provide some community nursing services, leaving much else offered by community and mixed trusts to these organizations. This 'cherry picking' of services which are relatively easy to run initially has been criticized, but given the relative inexperience of most PCGs, it may be wise that they do not provide more. PCGs are charged with allocating health care resources prudently and with improving the health of the communities they serve. This dual role is a departure from common practice for health authorities to be centres of excellence in evaluating illness services, and confining health improvement to poorly resourced, though enthusiastic health promotion departments.

PARTNERSHIP WORKING

PCGs and PCTs also represent a departure from previous practice in that they have a social service representative as a Board member. This should ensure that there is partnership working through the whole process of PCG planning and monitoring of services. Although there have been many discussions locally about the right level of social services' personnel on boards, when in doubt, local authorities have tended to put in more senior colleagues to give weight to the difficult decisions that have to be made.

A wider ring of partnership working is also being required of PCGs. As noted, the HImP documents set out both service issues and public health priorities for the health authority areas. Each HImP has to be agreed by all major stakeholders in the community. This has meant that, at senior level, agencies have had to consider the priorities of the health authority and match their own work plan against these priorities. In some places this has led to a more holistic view of local planning so that the myriad of schemes affecting a community (about 100 at present) may be coalesced into some rational process which recognizes the core responsibilities of the agencies but also plans partnership working and shared responsibilities for building a sustainable community. In some places this work has been galvanized by the HImP process; in others, the demise of the Joint Consultative Committee or the formation of a health action zone has been the trigger for a review of partnership working arrangements. Whatever the driver to these processes, the fact that all agencies have a common set of national priorities (partnership working, targeting those most needy, increasing consultation with the public etc.) has enabled closer working than was possible previously.

CLINICAL GOVERNANCE

What is the likelihood that HImPs and PCGs/PCTs can improve the care received by patients within the NHS? The previous government's quality agenda was expressed through clinical audit and corporate governance. This asked individuals (and, to a lesser extent, groups) to assess their own performance. This clinical audit (at first seen as a medical activity but soon embraced by the whole health community) was useful for motivated practitioners to prove to colleagues how services might be made to have better outcomes for patients or be more efficient of time or resources. Unfortunately, since the audit was practitioner-driven, there was little incentive to make these changes systemic and sometimes there was little connection in terms of decision-making between audit and the board room. During the 1990s, however, the notion of evidence-based practice gained currency. This school of thought argued that, contrary to common belief, much of the work of health professionals was not based on hard, irrefutable facts gained from clinical trials. Much, in fact, relied on shared tradition and experience. This did not come as a huge shock to nurses, used to the poor research base from which we derive our knowledge; nursing as art and science is not a new idea. However, in medicine this was more difficult to accept. The prime right of GPs and consultants to practise to their own standards had not been successfully challenged previously. This allowed for the notion that one of two ways of doing a hip replacement or treating hypertension was better, and the other worse, and therefore should not be practised.

The Labour government encouraged this drive to quality by structuring in changes to the NHS in a White Paper and subsequent guidance. *A First Class Service* (DOH, 1998a) produced a framework to ensure that PCGs and trusts pursued quality in the services they provided by making the quality of clinical care a Board-level indicator, along with corporate financial governance. It seems odd now to reflect that before this, chief executives were not (directly) responsible for the quality of clinical services offered in their hospitals/PCGs etc. – that was the domain of professionals. The case of the Bristol babies changed this irrevocably.

BRISTOL HEART SURGERY

In brief, the regional centre for heart surgery for the south-west of England is based at Bristol Royal Infirmary, where two supposedly eminent surgeons, James Wisheart and Janardan Dhasmana, were attempting arterial switch open heart surgery on children. Over the course of nearly 10 years they operated on 53 children with a death rate 40% higher than the national average for similar children with this condition (Gulland, 1998).

The question asked at the inquiry about this situation was: why did it take so long before anyone noticed these death rates were so high and how was it that the surgeons were not challenged more quickly? The answer emerging is, of course, very complex. The Chief Executive of the Trust, who was also a doctor, seemed reluctant to admit any criticism of the surgeons, believing their story of there being a steep 'learning curve' needed to reach success with their surgery. Clearly, the curve was not steep enough. There were those who did notice that practice was poor, indeed, one nurse made meticulous notes of the circumstances of the cases of children taken for heart surgery but she decided to leave the Trust rather than go through the trauma of challenging the doctors. Anecdotally, surrounding hospitals knew that the death rates were poor and chose to send children elsewhere for surgery. Finally, a respected anaesthetist, known for his background in clinical audit, blew the whistle and managed to bring high levels of attention to the dangerous practice of these doctors. For this, he lost his job in the Trust and has subsequently moved to Australia, believing that his actions would make it virtually impossible for him to find work here (Davidson, 1998). One of the two surgeons was banned from surgery; the other was told he would not be able to operate on children for three years. The Chief Executive lost his job.

It was no surprise that the non-health care press called for an end to self-regulation, believing that the relatively light nature of the sanctions placed on the doctors indicated a lack of will on the part of the General Medical Council to punish doctors seriously for malpractice. Others have welcomed the White Paper changes which would have ensured that a named person within the Trust would have been responsible for auditing the outcomes of these doctors' practice (Dickson, 1998).

The clinical governance strategy, due to be published by Easter 1998, was delayed as a result of the Bristol case. The resulting document had a strong message of challenge to the belief in self-regulation of doctors. Public horror in the wake of the murders of his patients by Dr Shipman (estimates vary from the 12 deaths for which he was convicted of murder to 150 potential victims) has only strengthened the hand of the Government. Whereas *A First Class Service* (DOH, 1998a) did not fundamentally question the right of professionals to call each other to account, it did create a national body, the National Institute for Clinical Excellence (NICE), charged with evaluating evidence for practices which may be questionable or have a dubious research base. Its choice of first-year priorities, including 'flu immunizations and tonsillectomy in children, will call to account medical practice. In addition, NICE described a national 'Offsted' for health, the Commission for Health Improvement (CHI), to inspect health bodies that do not come up to the standard expected of them. CHI is now being formed, so its effectiveness is as yet untested. At the centre of this national policy remains clinical governance. This requires the chief executives of health organizations to be accountable for the quality of clinical care in their sphere. This gives practitioners a vital route to the Board room which clinical audit lacked. It remains a peer-led activity, but with the possibility of Board-level blame, directors are now active in supporting systems to make certain services are of excellent quality.

Whether this high level of activity will succeed in changing the long-established right of practitioners (doctors are only one of many) who have seen it as their right and duty to decide personally on patterns of care, is yet to be seen. Certainly, Bristol proved an object lesson in this. However, there is much resistance to the influence of national guidance on the intimate choices made by practitioners for their patients.

There is also disquiet among many, nurses in particular, who question the basis for evaluation of some of the evidence. The research paradigm used by traditional medicine describes the 'gold standard' of evidence to be a randomized controlled trial. There is no doubt that many nursing interventions cannot be tested in this way, and further, it is very hard for these trials to reveal the health gain by public health interventions that might take five or even 30 years to show results. If NICE confines itself to randomized controlled trials, it will not be able to evaluate clearly much of real benefit (and some potential harm) within the NHS.

Implications for community nursing

What do these changes mean for nurses working in the community in the UK? We have had 10 years of politicians promising us a 'primary care-led NHS' with little to show for it. Power or resources have not been forthcoming – are these changes likely to improve that situation? The White Paper (*The New NHS – Modern and Dependable*; DOH, 1997b) described putting the '[community nurses] back in the driving seat in shaping local services in the future'. Has this promise been fulfilled?

An important consideration in any assessment of the implications of these changes for nursing is the fact that community nurses form an ageing work-force. Of district nurses, for example, nearly one-third are due to retire in the next 10–15 years – many more than are being trained (Audit Commission, 1999). This situation has led to a substantial skill mix as fully trained community nurses become fewer. The problem will become more acute in future years and any plan to expand the role and scope of community nursing must resolve this issue.

The most significant change has been the inclusion of two nurses on every PCG Board in England. This change requires nurses to be part of decision-making in these new bodies. At present, only commissioning decisions are being taken, but, in April 2000, 17 PCGs transferred to Trust status and became provider units. Nurses have a crucial role in forming these new orga-nizations, although with the strong representation of GPs on the Clinical Executive Boards of PCTs, their contribution may be diluted. What will nurses do with this new position? Will they be marginalized or empowered? Anecdotal evidence so far suggests that nurses have struggled to have the impact they hoped on PCG Boards. However, most would argue that these are early days and that as nurses gain experience in factual details and nego-tiation skills they will have much greater ability to influence the debate.

In the next few years PCTs will be at the heart of the NHS, and will be key to integrating community health services, general practice and social care to address the health of the local population and health inequalities.

PCTs will commission both primary and secondary services and provide community health services. It is essential for PCTs to have nurse representa-tion at both Board and executive level. Nurses are the link between patients and the Board. Community nurses can play a vital role as they identify health needs, help to implement local and national health improvement strategies and assess the effectiveness of interventions. It is the role of the PCT Board nurse to bring the public health perspective to the health agenda and incor-porate it into every community nurse's work.

The Royal College of Nursing (RCN, 1998) has stated that community nurses are well-placed to make a significant contribution to the commission-ing process. The RCN has identified several roles that Board-level nurses will need to develop. These are strategic thinker, political operator, practice devel-oper, organizational developer and manager of self. Nurses working in PCTs will need vision, leadership qualities and excellent communication skills.

Whatever their role in providing services, nurses are now uniquely placed to bring forward the debate on public and preventative health within main-stream services. Nurses and health visitors have talked about these issues for years, but now have an opportunity, with strong government backing, to allow these issues to become priorities within their organizations.

MAKING A DIFFERENCE – NURSING STRATEGY INTO THE NEXT 10 YEARS

In the summer of 1999, the government produced its strategy for nursing, *Making a Difference* (DOH, 1999b). This was more explicit about the new public health role for community nurses and envisaged health visitors, school nurses, occupational health nurses and infection control nurses as spearheading this agenda.

Health visitors

Health visitors are to have a family-centred public health role to improve health and tackle health inequalities. The government is encouraging them to work in new ways, to lead teams of nurses, nursery nurses and community workers. 'Skill-mix' is a new concept for most health visitors and Allen (2000) suggests that they are the most reluctant to delegate work. Although they understand themselves to have a population-based public health role, at present they still tend to focus on the individual and the family. They are being asked to undertake community profiling and health needs assessment and to focus on addressing the effect on health of poverty and social exclusion (DOH, 1999b). This work includes providing a public health role to groups such as the homeless, vulnerable children and their families, victims of domestic violence and socially isolated older people. This work has always been done; for example, two innovative health visitors working in Penwerris, the poorest and most deprived ward in the south-west, worked across professional boundaries to achieve real change in a ghetto estate. The estate had a history of escalating violence, fear and tension. Previously, no social activities took place on the estate. The health visitors started a tenants' and residents' association, and then went on to develop a parents and toddler group, parenting courses, neighbourhood watch and after school clubs in response to identified needs. There were positive health outcomes: the crime rate was reduced by 50%; the number of children on the Child Protection Register came down from 23 in 1995 to eight in 1999; the children's SAT results improved by 100%, and the number of patients treated for post-natal depression came down from 18 in 1995, to four in 1999 (Stutley and Trenoweth, 1999). *Making a Difference* (DOH, 1999b) requires this way of working to become much more common. This public health role has been prominent in areas which have attracted funding, latterly those in health action zones and those who bid successfully for the first round of Sure Start money. The latter supports young families in deprived areas to build parenting capacity within communities, improving the chances for young children to grow up healthy and to be able to take up opportunities offered them. It is not clear whether in areas where no new money exists, health visitors will be able to make the changes required in *Saving Lives* (DOH, 1999a) and *Making a Difference* (DOH, 1999b).

School nurses

Making a Difference (DOH, 1999b) also acknowledges the diverse role of school nurses and sees them as pivotal, like health visitors, in delivering the public health agenda. They, too, would lead teams and work in partnership with health visitors and teachers to support policies such as the healthy schools

initiative. Nationally, we have the highest rate of teenage conception in western Europe (Social Exclusion Unit, 1999) and bringing this down is a key target
of the government. School nurses are charged with supporting young people
in accessing sexual health and contraceptive advice. Other priorities for
school nurses are improving parenting skills, working with excluded children
and smoking cessation initiatives.

Midwives

Making a Difference (DOH, 1999b) visualizes an expanded role for midwives,
and for them to play a bigger role in the government's public health strategy.
Midwives are being encouraged to work in partnership with health visitors
and school nurses to provide care and advice on all aspects of women's
health. They are also asked to play a stronger role in health promotion to give
advice about issues such as smoking, exercise and diet.

General practice nurses

Of all nurses in the community, the changes arguably offer general practice
nurses the greatest challenge. Recent educational developments have meant
that they can now gain a degree-level qualification in 'General Practice
Nursing'. Others have taken a different route and are studying to be nurse
practitioners (along with some other community nurses). Many general practice nurses now have great responsibilities for the management of chronic disease and health promotion within general practice. Indeed, although they
were denied the first round of nurse prescribing, general practice nurses now
have effective control of large groups of patients, including those with
chronic diseases such as diabetes and asthma. Many are now on PCG Boards,
although not in they numbers they might wish, yet despite this, many general
practice nurses still feel isolated working as they do in the small businesses
of general practice. Many work without sufficient investment in their clinical
and professional development, with inadequate clinical supervision, and
lacking access to rights of union representation and the same pay and conditions enjoyed by the rest of their community nursing colleagues. Many of the
latter still see general practice nurses as under the heavy influence of GPs,
although PCGs are reducing this perception. PCTs offer the chance for all
community nurses to be employed by the same organization which may dissolve this artificial barrier.

Opportunities for general practice nurses look promising. For example,
they will play a leading role in improving community cardiac services under
the new national service framework for coronary heart disease (DOH, 2000a).
There is evidence to suggest practice nurse-led heart clinics in general practice have improved aspirin use, blood pressure, lipid management, physical
activity and diet (Campbell *et al.*, 1998). The interface between district nursing
and general practice nursing is under scrutiny (DOH, 1999b); the disciplines
are closely related and now there is an opportunity to explore joint potential,
and share workload skills and knowledge.

District nurses

The Audit Commission (1999) surveyed all NHS Trusts providing district nursing services (91% response) and found that with demand for district nursing care, the potential effectiveness of district nurses was not being utilized. The Audit Commission highlighted the need for clear referral criteria, a method of caseload management that promotes safe and effective practice, an equitable out-of-hours service, the need for standardized documentation guidelines, continuing education and training and the development of regular clinical supervision and audit.

The role of the district nurse is changing in response to hospital utilization. England has fewer general and acute beds per head of population than many other countries (DOH, 2000b). Alongside this, the average length of hospital stay is falling and bed occupancy is rising (DOH, 2000b). So, with fewer beds, more patients are being treated and are being discharged home sooner. Many trusts and PCGs are investing in intermediate care services such as rapid response teams and developing a 24-hour district nursing service (for example, the Bolton Model cited by the Audit Commission, 1999). The emergence of rapid response teams has assisted in preventing hospital admissions and facilitating early discharges, especially for elderly patients (Audit Commission, 1999). They have enabled treatments such as the administration of blood transfusions, treatment of deep vein thromboses and intravenous antibiotics to be given in patients' own homes.

District nursing was not identified as having a major public health role in the implementation of *Saving Lives* (DOH, 1999a). However, Wilson (2000) advocates that district nurses are in a key position to become involved in the expert patient initiative. The government is encouraging a self-care initiative for individuals suffering from chronic illness or disability (DOH, 1999a), and it is this group of patients that district nurses spend much time caring for and educating.

Nurse consultants

A key component of *Making a Difference* (DOH, 1999b) is the appointment of nurse consultants. It is intended that these posts should improve services and quality and strengthen nursing leadership. Irrespective of the field of practice, setting or service in which it is based, each post should be structured around four core functions that exemplify the role (NHSE, 1999):

- An expert practice function.
- A professional leadership and consultancy function.
- An education, training and development function.
- A practice and service development, research and evaluation function.

All consultant nurse posts will be embedded in clinical practice and at least 50% of their time will be spent in working directly with patients, clients or communities. Nurse consultants are being established to provide new career opportunities for experienced and expert nurses who previously left practice-based posts to advance their careers and improve their earnings.

Nurses managing a personal medical service pilot or walk-in centre are possible models for the consultant nurse. Forester (1999) argues the case for those
with a high level of generalist knowledge to qualify as nurse consultants, in
the same way that GPs are considered to be at consultant status because of the
levels of knowledge and skills needed to be a generalist.

NEW ROLES FOR COMMUNITY NURSES

Nurses have taken up new roles as changes have taken place in the NHS. For
example, personal medical service pilots (previously known as 'Primary Care
Act' pilot sites) enable health authorities to relax the very strict rules around
the running of general practice – the Red Book. In areas of greater deprivation, in particular for the homeless and those from ethnic minorities, personal
medical service centres can offer health care structured very differently from
present primary care. Some of the most innovative of these centres are run by
nurses. The nurses manage the services, offer nurse practitioner-level care
and employ doctors to give medical care when required. They have been
successful in raising the standard of care received by these groups and in
establishing successful direct employment of doctors in primary care. Whilst
it is not envisaged by the government that this will become standard practice
across the country, it does show that the structure of general practice can be
successfully challenged by nurses (Forester, 1999).

A second key new role for nurses is in the new NHS Direct service. This is
a nurse-led 24-hour helpline that could become a central gateway to health
care, hitherto the traditional role of the GP. Not all GPs are comfortable with
this new service. The feeling of unease was expressed at the GPs' annual conference in June 1999 when a third of delegates voted to scrap this scheme.
Critics believe that NHS Direct will increase demand on GPs and accident
and emergency departments (Florin and Rosen, 1999).

In some areas, such as Nottingham, GP opposition has been minimized by
the linkage of NHS Direct and out-of-hours GP co-operatives. All the calls to
GP co-operatives go via NHS Direct, are triaged by the nurses and home
visits arranged. In Nottingham only 46% of calls were referred back to GPs
(O'Dowd, 1999).

NHS Direct now covers most of England and initial evaluation shows that
pressure on accident and emergency services was less in some areas covered
by NHS Direct, but as yet there is not enough evidence to measure the impact
of the scheme on the NHS; however, patient satisfaction levels are high
(Sheffield University, 1998).

Nurse practitioner

Nowhere is the tension between nursing and medicine so apparent as in
the emerging role of the nurse practitioner. Some nurses perceive the development as the medicalization of nursing, whereas some doctors are wary
they may lose their power within the medical profession. The term 'nurse
practitioner' has given rise to much confusion and debate in the past and

their development has been hampered by a lack of regulation. The Royal College of Nursing (RCN, 1997) sees the key feature of their role as a nurse who will assess patients' needs, prescribe and interpret diagnostic tests, diagnose and, where possible, treat patients. There are many community nurses who would argue that they do all this already, and that the extra training of the nurse practitioner is unnecessary, given the very high levels of skill available among community nurses. However, the unique contribution of nurse practitioners in practice is to see patients who do not neatly fall into the categories seen by present community nurses for a much wider range of conditions than most nurses see at present.

With the shortfall in GP recruitment and the drive to a cost-efficient primary-led NHS, there will be increased pressure for doctors to relinquish some of their clinical work to nurse practitioners. At present many operate inside general practice, in personal medical services sites and other more innovative primary care settings. The prescribing changes hoped for (DOH, 1999c) could enhance and extend their role. All these initiatives could place the nurse practitioner in a position to take up a generalist nurse consultant post.

Nurse prescribing

Community nurse prescribing is now well-established and has extended their scope of practice and helped to speed up treatment. This has been achieved after many years of lobbying by nursing unions. Unfortunately, the scope of the nursing formulary is at present quite limited. However, the Rubicon has been crossed and the formulary can only widen in subsequent years. Possible areas for this include care of minor ailments in children (to health visitors and school nurses) and the care of the elderly who have a range of minor ailments (to district nurses). However, prescribing by nurses on the basis of group protocols has taken place in hospitals and primary care with no clear basis in law (Dimond, 2000). The final report of the Crown review (DOH, 1999c) recommended that there should be two types of prescriber, an independent and a dependent prescriber. An independent prescriber is responsible for the initial assessment of the patient and for devising the treatment plan, with the authority to prescribe as part of that plan. A dependent prescriber would be able to prescribe within agreed clinical guidelines or an individual patient treatment plan approved by an independent prescriber.

The government has cited nurses who manage patients with asthma or diabetes, or those who work in walk-in centres as being suitable candidates for this role. These proposals will ensure there is a clear, satisfactory basis for prescribing and supply of medication that has hitherto taken place under group protocols.

Conclusion

Nursing in the community has been characterized as the role that often promises far more than it delivers. The new Labour government is no different to many others in suggesting that community nurses could have expanded roles in commissioning, public health and clinical practice. There are some structural changes which give substantial hope that some of the changes promised may come to fruition. The proof of the changes will certainly be judged by how well nurses have been able to adapt their services to meet the health needs of the most-excluded members of the population. It remains to be seen, given the existing population of nurses and the constraints of tradition and finance, how successful they will prove to be.

There are certainly many opportunities opening up for community nurses. Nurse-led projects flourish as never before. Alan Milburn described how he saw nursing developing in a modernized NHS. He wishes to use the full potential of nurses in order to free up doctors. It is debatable whether the biggest emphasis is the reduction in junior doctors' hours or a new nursing strategy.

As the largest professional group within the NHS, the contribution of community nurses, midwives and health visitors cannot be underestimated, and we need to work in collaboration with colleagues from other disciplines in delivering the health agenda.

References

Allen, D. (2000) The vision thing. *Community Practitioner*, 72: 461–3.

Atkin, K. and Lunt, N. (1995) *Nurses count: a national census of practice nurses.* York: Social Policy Research Unit, University of York.

Audit Commission. (1999) *First assessment: a review of district nursing services in England and Wales.* London: Audit Commission.

Campbell, N.C., Ritchie, L.D. and Thain, J. (1998) Secondary prevention in CHD: a randomised trial of nurse led clinics in primary care. *Heart*, 80: 447–52.

Davidson, L. (1998) Alarm unheard or unheeded? *Health Service Journal*, 108: 514–15.

Department of Health (DOH). (1992) *Health of the nation.* London: DOH.

Department of Health (DOH). (1997a) *Report into the inequalities in health (the Acheson Report).* London: The Stationery Office.

Department of Health (DOH). (1997b) *The new NHS – modern and dependable.* London: The Stationery Office.

Department of Health (DOH). (1998a) *A first class service.* London: DOH.

Department of Health (DOH). (1998b) *Our healthier nation: a contract for health.* London: The Stationery Office.

Department of Health (DOH. (1999a) *Our healthier nation: saving lives.* London: DOH.

Department of Health (DOH). (1999b) *Making a difference – strengthening the nursing, midwifery and health visiting contribution to health and healthcare.* London: DOH.

Department of Health (DOH). (1999c) *Review of prescribing, supply and administration medicines final report (shaping the Crown Report).* London: DOH.

Department of Health (DOH). (2000a) *Modern standards and service models. Coronary heart disease national service framework.* London: DOH.

Department of Health (DOH). (2000b) *Future NHS: long term planning for and related services consultation document on the national beds inquiry – supporting analysis.* London: DOH.

Dickson, N. (1998) Editorial – body politic. *Nursing Times*, 94: 26.

Dimond, B. (2000) Legal issues arising in community nursing 5: Nurse prescribing. *Journal of Community Nursing*, 5: 186–9.

Florin, D. and Rosen, R. (1999) Evaluating NHS Direct. Early findings raise questions expanding the service. *British Medical Journal*, 319: 5–6.

Forester, S. (1999) Nurse consultants in primary care. *Community Practitioner*, 72: 365–7.

Gulland, A. (1998) Heartfelt concerns. *Nursing Times*, 94: 12–13.

NHS Executive. (1999) *HSC (1999/217) nurse, midwife and health visitor consultants – posts and making appointments.* London: NHSE.

O'Dowd, A. (1999) Ringing the changes. *Nursing Times*, 95: 26–9.

Royal College of Nursing. (1997) *Statement on the role and scope of the nurse practitioner.* London: RCN.

Royal College of Nursing. (1998) *The new primary care groups: the knowledge and skills needed to make them a success.* London: RCN.

Sheffield University. (1998) *Evaluation of NHS Direct first wave sites. First interim report to the DOH.* Sheffield: Sheffield University.

Stutley, H. and Trenoweth, P. (1999) *The Beacon project – Falmouth, Cornwall.* Cornwall Healthcare Trust, unpublished.

The public health agenda – can it really be part of community nursing?

2

Carolyn Mason

Introduction

This chapter examines a key dimension of community nursing – public health, asking a central question: can the public health agenda really be part of community nursing? The chapter begins with an analysis of the term 'public health' and its associated policy agenda. The initial setting will be the global and European context for public health. This is followed by a sharper focus on public health in the UK within the political framework of devolution and evolving primary care delivery systems. Perhaps most importantly, the chapter then takes a critical look at the connections between community nursing and public health, bearing in mind the tension that often exists between primary care and public health and the constraints on community nurses who wish to work to a more explicit public health remit. Models for delivering and enhancing the public health role in community nursing are offered, and the chapter concludes with an assessment of the potential for the public health agenda to integrate in a meaningful way with community nursing practice.

What is public health?

Popular notions of 'public health' tend to concentrate on 'drains and sewers', sanitation and infectious diseases. An epidemiological view of public health might focus on immunization, communicable disease outbreaks and lifestyle issues associated, for example, with heart disease, whereas sociologists might be more likely to emphasize poverty and the socio-economic conditions that impact on health. Add to this a growing concern about the effect of environmental influences on the health of the public, and it becomes clear that the term 'public health' can become all-encompassing to the point of losing its working value.

A review of the literature on public health reveals a range of definitions, some of which are listed below:

... the committee* defines public health as fulfilling society's interest in assuring conditions in which people can be healthy. Public health is distinguished from health care by its focus on community wide concerns – the public interest – rather than the interests of particular individuals or groups. Its aim is to generate organized community effort to address public concerns about health by applying scientific and technological change.

(Institute of Medicine, 1988: 1)

... the science and art of preventing disease, prolonging life and promoting health through the organised efforts of society

(Acheson, 1988: 16)

... a collective view of the health needs and health care of a population rather than an emphasis on an individual perspective. A central component of this collective approach is an emphasis on a partnership at all stages and levels of the public health process. This means partnership with communities and clients within them as well as partnerships across and between professional groups. Teamwork is an essential prerequisite to effective public health work.

(RCN, 1994: 1)

A number of points can be noted. For example, the definitions tend to emphasize the social, rather than individual, effort required to achieve public health. They are mainly statements of intention, referring to aims and process and this arguably indicates the difficulties associated with determining the concept of public health, as distinct from how to do public health. Not least, it may be salutary to note that the first definition is from the US Institute of Medicine – its emphasis on 'organized community effort' belies easy stereotyping of that profession's reliance on 'the medical model'.

The definitions derive from two distinct orientations and knowledge bases as indicated in Figure 2.1.

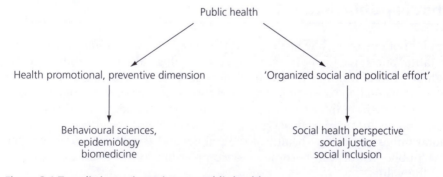

Public health

Health promotional, preventive dimension ← → 'Organized social and political effort'

Behavioural sciences, epidemiology biomedicine

Social health perspective social justice social inclusion

Figure 2.1 Two distinct orientations to public health

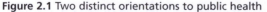

*The Public Health Committee of the US Institute of Medicine.

It is asserted here that there is merit in each approach. Although it may be dangerous to overemphasize individual health promotion in situations where people are powerless to adopt recommended behaviours, knowledge about beneficial behaviour change can be empowering for those with the motivation and wherewithal to alter their lifestyle. At the same time, the profound effect of socio-economic and environmental influences on health must never be forgotten. Even in the richest countries in Europe, 'the better-off live several years longer and have fewer illnesses and disabilities than the poor. Poverty is the biggest risk factor for health' (WHO, 1998: Section 14).

In summary, it is apparent that there is no single definition, conceptualiza-tion or operational framework for public health. 'Public health' is not an entity that can easily be isolated from the totality of social and health services and it includes a wide range of political, social, environmental and health promotional activity. Nevertheless, it is possible to identify recurring themes from the literature and policy documents in terms of the aim, action and underpinning values of public health, as outlined below.

AIM

The aim of public health is to make people, i.e. populations and individuals, healthy or, as expressed by the World Health Organization (WHO) (WHO, 1998) 'to add human comfort'. The implication is that health can be broadly conceived as incorporating physical, mental and social well-being, as defined by the WHO (WHO, 1948). The intention is to prevent disease, prolong life and promote health (Acheson, 1988) and this is often expressed in terms of a dual purpose with a positive dimension (to promote health) and a preventive dimension (to prevent illness).

ACTION

To achieve health in populations and in individuals, the consensus appears to be that public health action is more than medical care and involves (a) socio-environmental measures to create the conditions for people to attain and maintain health and (b) health promotion to encourage individual responsi-bility for healthy lifestyles. Taken together, these socio-environmental and health promotion measures, as reported in the literature, can be subdivided into four levels:

- Government policy, for example, in relation to sanitation and hygiene, action to reduce poverty, air pollution and road accidents, etc.
- Health service measures, such as immunization programmes, commis-sioning services for health improvement, information systems and methods of evaluation.
- Action at local level, key to which is the involvement and participation of communities. This includes community assessment and community health profiling by community nurses, and community development work.

- Individually focused health promotion, such as health education by community nurses on a one-to-one basis or in groups, clinics in health centres where there is a health promotion content and much of the work of midwives with antenatal women and health visitors with mothers and children.

UNDERPINNING VALUES

There is marked convergence in thinking on the values that underpin public health. These can be listed as follows:

- Equity and social inclusion.
- Participation, collaboration and community empowerment.
- Social justice/health as a human right and, to a lesser extent, accountability of agencies for identifying public health improvement measures with emphasis on high standards and quality assurance.

It may be concluded that public health aims to make people healthy through organized social effort and health promotion, centred on principles of equity, participation and social justice. A working definition of public health for nursing, therefore, could be that public health is *organized social and political effort, and health promotion for the benefit of populations, families and individuals.*

The strategic drive for public health

The public health agenda has been consistently promoted by the WHO at global and European levels. It may be useful first to outline the European region targets for public health, as the wider framework within which community nurses in the UK practice (Table 2.1).

The WHO *Health 21* targets (WHO, 1998) represent a composite of the public health themes already highlighted: equity, healthy public policy and multisectoral responsibility for health. A lifespan approach is evident in targets 3–5 and this may be especially useful for community nurses for whom a sequential 'cradle to grave' orientation is familiar. The 'settings approach' to health action also has resonance with community nursing, arguing for joint planning to achieve more healthy lives in the home, pre-school, school and work environments. For example, it is recommended that pupils, teachers and parents – working with local communities and supported by their health advisors – should together design and evaluate health interventions such as smoking-free activities involving all three groups. This approach dovetails easily with the CPHVA/QNI/RCN (2000) Strategy for school nursing practice. *School Nursing within the Public Health Agenda*. ogether, the two reports develop a challenging, forward-looking public health orientation for school nursing in the UK, and form a good example of the integration of European WHO policy and more localized UK strategy.

Table 2.1   *Health 21* targets for health policy in European countries (WHO, 1998)

1	Closing the health gap between countries
2	Closing the health gap within countries
3	A healthy start in life (supportive family policies)
4	Health of young people (policies to reduce child abuse, accidents, drug use, unwanted pregnancies)
5	Healthy ageing (policies to improve health, self-esteem and independence before dependence emerges)
6	Improving mental health
7	Reducing communicable diseases
8	Reducing non-communicable diseases
9	Reducing injury from violence and accidents
10	A healthy and safe physical environment
11	Healthier living (fiscal, agricultural and retail policies that increase the availability of and access to and consumption of vegetables and fruits)
12	Reducing harm from alcohol, drugs and tobacco
13	A settings approach to health action (homes should be designed and built in a manner conducive to sustainable health and the environment)
14	Multisectoral responsibility for health
15	An integrated health sector and much stronger emphasis on primary care
16	Managing for quality of care using the European health for all indicators to focus on outcomes and compare the effectiveness of different inputs
17	Equitable and sustainable funding of health services
18	Developing human resources (educational programmes for providers and managers based on the principles of the health for all policy)
19	Research and knowledge: health programmes based on scientific evidence
20	Mobilizing partners for health (engaging the media/TV/internet)
21	Policies and strategies for health for all – national, targeted policies based on health for all

Within the UK, there has been a regeneration of interest in public health as an outcome of socio-economic and environmental influences, particularly since the Labour government came into power in 1997. This resurgence is manifested in public health strategies for England (DOH, 1999a), Wales (DOH Wales, 1998), Scotland (DOH Scotland, 1998) and Northern Ireland (DHSSPS, 2000) with the respective devolutionary governing bodies espousing public health, in varying degree, as an important political issue.

Analysis of the public health strategies for the four countries of the UK reveals marked similarities in terms of approach and target areas. All emphasize the importance of tackling the root causes of ill health, i.e. poverty, unemployment and poor environment/air pollution. Low educational achievement and inadequate housing are also highlighted in the Scottish strategy. The four regions place heart disease, cancer and mental health as primary targets for health improvement and pinpoint smoking, poor nutrition and alcohol consumption as major lifestyle factors with a health impact. Proposed strategies for achieving health targets vary somewhat between regions and include, for example, health impact assessments*, health action zones, sustainable development policies and tackling social exclusion.

Towards public health practice

This section looks briefly at public health practice in the context of the broader political and health arena. It is important to appreciate that this is the international public health framework within which community nurses work. Clarification of this agenda is essential in order to test the assertion that the public health agenda can or cannot be part of community nursing.

In 1986, the WHO held its first International Conference on Health Promotion in Ottawa, Canada. The outcome was the *Ottawa Charter for Health Promotion* (WHO, 1986), which translates the principles of public health into five action points, as shown in Table 2.2.

Table 2.2 The *Ottawa Charter* (WHO, 1986) action points for public health

Building **healthy public policy**, e.g. legislation that restricts smoking in public places
Re-orienting the health services to advocate for health and to achieve a greater balance between health promotion and curative services
Creating supportive environments – encouraging **environmental measures** which improve health, e.g. better, affordable housing, innovative transport policies, pollution control and recycling opportunities
Strengthening **community action** by incorporating community development approaches into health promotion interventions so that communities are empowered to take control and improve their health collectively
Developing **personal skills** by consulting individuals to identify their needs, involving them in the process of planning and evaluation of health promotion programmes to make them relevant and accessible

*Assessment of the impact of all major policies, for example, on housing, transport and education, on health.

Within the WHO's European region, four main strategies for action have been identified:

- *Multisectoral strategies* to tackle the determinants of health, ensuring the use of health impact assessment.
- *Health-outcome-driven programmes* and investments for health development and clinical care.
- *Integrated family- and community-oriented primary health care.*
- *A participatory health development process* that involves relevant partners for health at home, school and work and at local community and country levels, and that promotes joint decision-making, implementation and accountability (WHO, 1998: 9).

Can community nurses in the UK take on this vast agenda? Can it be asked realistically that community nurses build policy and reorientate the health service? To what extent can they influence environmental measures such as better housing and cheaper public transport? Perhaps a more practical question would be, what is the extent to which community nurses *contribute* to the agenda, accepting that different levels of contribution may be acceptable and appropriate. As community nurses, we might argue that we are stronger in developing personal skills, as described above by the WHO, but do we really consult mothers, schoolchildren and elderly people to find out their priorities, planning with them the steps to take? Community development might feature strongly in the rhetoric of community nursing, but how often, in practice, do we meet with community leaders so that we can complement each other's work to improve local conditions? The issue of integrated family *and* community-orientated primary health care is crucial, and may involve some tension for community nurses between primary care and public health agendas. This and other issues will be picked up in subsequent sections, which focus specifically on community nursing and public health.

Community nursing and public health practice

If we accept that public health practice derives from the WHO and the *Ottawa Charter* (WHO, 1986) guidance on multisectoral working, community action and collaborative personal skills enhancement, we can make a strong case in support of nursing involvement in that agenda. With respect to multisectoral working, nursing is key to public health. Perhaps more than any other social, health or medical workers, nurses cross the boundaries between public, voluntary and private health and social care sectors. For example, nurses form the largest proportion of the workforce in the acute health care sector. They are central to the delivery of care in private nursing and residential homes, to caregiving in the privacy of family and home settings, while also working in the independent school sector and occupational health departments of private industry.

Thus, nurses form a key link between sectors in the provision of health promotion, care and treatment. Nursing activity spans the full spectrum of public health action, from, for example, meningococcal and influenza immunization to community empowerment. Nurses working at government, Health Authority/Board and Trust levels have the potential to make links between departments and organizations such as employment, housing, transport and environment. One illustration is the allocation of funding for Surestart projects – a major government initiative – where community nurses have been actively involved with representatives from education, city councils and others in submitting proposals and leading early years projects.

Moving beyond intersectoral to interagency working, it is notable that, increasingly, nurses appear to be taking on leadership roles in the voluntary sector. For example, in Northern Ireland the Director of the well-developed and influential Community Development and Health Network is a nurse. Similarly, the Director of Women Against Violence (WAVE) – a voluntary movement with a major role in post-conflict situation trauma management – is a nurse. This is in addition to crucial roles, for instance in the hospice movement and Marie Curie, and specialist voluntary organizations for people with disabilities, diabetes and other special needs. Such posts embody the cross-sectoral, partnership spirit of public health, which is not about professional boundaries but rather about imaginative, productive linking of skills, at all levels, for public benefit. Nurse-led public health projects with local communities and targeted populations (travellers, women working in prostitution, for example) serve to reinforce the point that community nursing skills are well-tailored to public health work.

The importance of community nurses as a source of insight into local culture and health beliefs should not be underestimated. Community nurses often gain the trust of local people. Over time, they 'know' communities intimately, and are therefore crucial informants for public health needs assessments. They are in a key position both to provide information relating to health needs and to influence health behaviour.

Further arguments can be made in support of the contention that the public health agenda is part of community nursing. For example, a major research study of all nurses working in community settings* in Northern Ireland (Poulton et al., 2000) concluded that there was a high level of public health activity within community nursing practice. In the research study, 'public health activity' was considered to have five dimensions as identified by Holman (1992) (Table 2.3).

Overall, community nurses were found to be most active in the areas of health education and primary, secondary and tertiary prevention. Figure 2.2 illustrates public health activity by job title. Differences between disciplines were revealed with health visitors reporting most activity in the general area of community-orientated public health. The lowest levels of activity, for all disciplines, were in community empowerment, health protection and healthy public policy and results showed a lack of confidence in developing, securing funding for and evaluating public health projects.

*This includes health visitors, district nurses, practice nurses, school nurses, community mental health nurses, community learning disability nurses, treatment room nurses, midwives, staff nurses, specialist nurses (e.g. in diabetes, continence, etc.) and 'others' such as managers and team leaders.

Table 2.3   Holman's (1992) typography of public health movements

Type of public health	Characteristics
Health protection	Enforced regulation of human behaviour to protect the health of individuals and populations. For example, fluoridation of water supplies, compulsory seatbelt-wearing in cars. Stresses collectivism at the expense of individual autonomy.
Preventative medicine	Primary, secondary and tertiary level preventative interventions. Secondary prevention, for example, aims to halt the progression of an existing disease, e.g. cervical screening and mammography programmes. Criticisms relate to questionable clinical and cost-effectiveness.
Health education	Provision of learning experiences that facilitate voluntary behaviour change for health improvement. Recent emphasis has shifted from passive listening to active learner participation and a wider range of methods, e.g. media, billboard advertising. This approach carries with it a risk of victim-blaming and possible use by politicians to divert attention away from healthy public policy.
Healthy public policy	Seeks to create a social, economic and physical environment that helps people make healthy choices. This approach derives from concern about the impact of poverty on health and is aligned with the WHO Healthy Cities project and the *Ottawa Charter*. Health is viewed as the responsibility of all policy-makers and includes, for example, pricing policies on tobacco and alcohol and access for disabled people to public buildings. Concerns relate to practical effectiveness and the risk of system-blaming rather than victim-blaming.
Community empowerment	Centres on community participation in decision-making. There is little emphasis on professional expertise because the notion that the 'expert knows best' is implicitly denied. Critiques point to inadequately informed decisions without reference to the 'wider picture' and a lack of coherence that militates against major social reform.

Although it is important to emphasize that public health activity is part of all branches of community nursing, a forceful argument can be made in support of the notion that public health is integrated in particular with the work of one specialism, health visiting. The principles of health visiting (CETHV, 1977; Twinn and Cowley, 1992) were originally written in 1977; they are grounded in public health and have endured through major changes in health service delivery over the decades. These principles are shown in Table 2.4.

The principles demonstrate the close alignment between the public health agenda and the basis of health visiting practice. They indicate that health visitors are community-based nurse specialists who develop a range of interventions tailored to assessed need while using local community knowledge to influence policy. Under UKCC community specialist health practice, health visitors are called 'public health nurses'. However, while the title and the

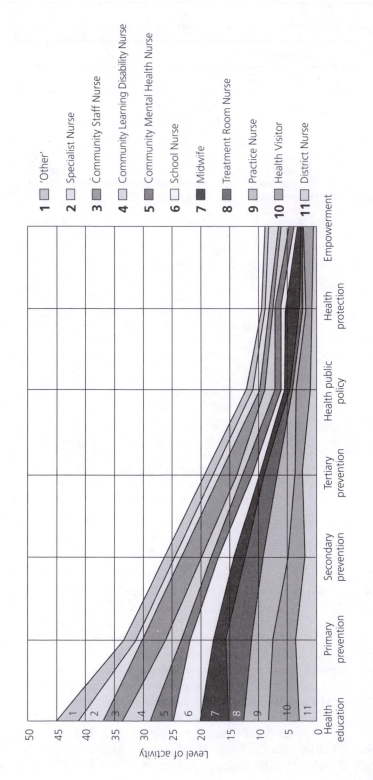

Figure 2.2 Public health activity by job title (source: Poulton *et al.*, 2000)

Table 2.4   The principles of health visiting (CETHV, 1977)

The search for health needs
Stimulation of the awareness of health needs
The influence on policies affecting health
The facilitation of health-enhancing activities

principles may reflect a professional aspiration to public health practice, constraints in the primary care setting may compromise the professional goal. This will now be discussed with relation to health visiting and community nursing in general.

Challenges to the community nursing contribution to public health practice

In spite of the positive public health policy context, there are challenges to the community nursing capacity to work to a public health agenda.

It is acknowledged internationally that a distinction exists between primary health care and primary care. Primary health care is the WHO approach to addressing inequalities in health status (Baum *et al.*, 1992) and it has been argued that primary health care equates to public health (Sandhu, 1996). In contrast, primary care is a more limited concept involving first contact medical services (MacDonald, 1992; Sandhu, 1996). In the UK, primary care means care centred on the primary health care team, including the core GP practice team, plus pharmacy, optometry and dental services, community nursing, the professions allied to medicine (e.g. physiotherapy, podiatry), health promotion, direct social services, home care, day care and social support services (SHSSB, 1997). A plethora of models for the delivery of primary care have been tested throughout the UK, including primary care groups, total purchasing pilots, mental health pilots, maternity pilots, personal medical services pilots and primary care commissioning pilots. Since April 2000 in England, a number of primary care groups (PCGs) have coalesced into primary care Trusts (PCTs) to commission and provide services, run community hospitals and community health services, employ the necessary staff and own property (DOH England, 2000a).

The key principles of primary care have tended to focus on the quality and efficiency of service delivery. For example, *The New NHS: Modern, Dependable* (DOH, 1997) identified the following underpinning principles for primary care:

- Consistent national standards.
- Devolved responsibility.
- Partnership working between local authorities and trusts.
- Improved efficiency by cutting bureaucracy.
- Focus on excellence.
- Openness and accountability.

More recently, *The NHS Plan* (DOH England, 2000b) calls for structural improvements, e.g. modernization, of GP premises and the bringing together of health and social care into care Trusts; efficiencies, e.g. quality-based contracts for GPs, and reduced waiting times; and the development of professional functions, e.g. more nurse consultants, and an extension to the number of nurses able to prescribe medicines.

In summary, primary care and public health have two discrete but overlapping agendas. Put starkly, primary care is health-focused – in particular on general medical services – with an emphasis on how the NHS works, while public health is about achieving equity through integrated government policy, intersectoral effort and community involvement. Community nurses, and perhaps especially health visitors, can be caught between the two. The greater volume of the health visiting service may be contracted to GPs/PCGs. General practice priorities are defined by the GP Contract, with a concentration on meeting identified targets, for example on immunizations and screening. This tends to preclude the health needs assessment and community empowerment type of public health work upon which health visitors may wish to focus. Although the importance of the preventive, screening and biomedical aspects of public health are fully acknowledged, unfortunately, an exclusive focus on these areas has resulted in a devaluation of community-based public health, with non-renewal, by GPs, of contracts for health visiting services in some parts of England.

Other barriers to effective public health practice include large caseloads (CPHVA, 1999) and lack of management support. Poulton *et al.* (2000) found that community nurses in Northern Ireland perceived their employers (Trusts) as responsive to change and having organizational commitment to public health, but weak on providing practical assistance with new ideas and leadership for public health practice. The most immediate barrier to public health activity in practice, for many health visitors, is the predominance of crisis, reactive and child protection work.

Overcoming the challenges: capacity building for public health practice

A major strategic drive is currently underway to build the capacity of nursing to contribute to the public health agenda. In 1998, the European Chief Nursing Officers (CNOs), including the four UK-based CNOs, determined that Member States should strengthen the nursing contribution to public health in their own countries by:

- Agreeing strategically the nursing contribution to public health.
- Analysing the public health agenda.
- Putting in place action plans to deliver the nursing contribution.
- Stimulating leadership in public health (CNO Report, 1998).

This has subsequently been reinforced in the *Munich Declaration* (WHO, 2000) which acknowledges the 'formidable' public health challenge in the context of rising consumer expectations, growing elderly populations, increases in certain preventable lifestyle-related diseases, infectious diseases and mental illness, along with greater poverty in some sections of society and increasing family breakdown. The European Ministers of Health, as signatories to the *Munich Declaration*, articulated explicitly their support for public health, health promotion and community development role-enhancement in nursing.

Initiatives are underway in Scotland, Northern Ireland, England and Wales to work on the CNO agenda. Two resulting reports (Poulton *et al.*, 2000; Scottish Executive 2000) highlight a range of strategic and professional themes and recommendations to enhance the contribution of nurses, midwives and health visitors to public health. It is noteworthy that although the Scotland and Northern Ireland reviews used different approaches – a consultation exercise and a census survey, respectively— the issues and recommendations are similar, covering strategic, organizational and professional measures to strengthen the nursing contribution to public health.

STRATEGIC MEASURES TO STRENGTHEN THE NURSING CONTRIBUTION TO PUBLIC HEALTH

The Scottish review points out that most nursing work on public health is *ad hoc* and marginal; therefore a more strategic approach is required including workforce planning, a pro-active approach to the deployment of nursing skills and continuing professional development.

A potentially significant strategic measure would be the reformulation of service-level agreements to create the necessary flexibility for creative community public health work. Many health authorities/health and social services Boards continue to use counts of client contacts as the contract currency for health visiting. The mismatch between contact counting and the development of innovative public health initiatives is well-recognized (Mason, 1995) and repeated calls have been made for service-level agreements that focus on good practice and outcomes. This must be a professional strategic priority and community nurses need to maximize opportunities to influence PCG and PCT contracts to allow for flexible working in response to identified need.

A number of contract frameworks have been suggested in the policy literature. In 1994, for example, the Department of Health produced a framework for school nursing service contracts under the headings 'Health of the nation targets', 'Professional involvement' and 'Opportunities for health-promoting activities' as shown in Table 2.5.

This framework is flexible enough to allow for public health activity across the spectrum of preventive, policy and community-based practice while permitting role enhancement as strategic and professional priorities shift. Arguably, the framework should also incorporate identification of local priorities based on assessed need or local health improvement plans and, in addition, outcome measures or at least some form of evaluation. Standards and performance measures could also be included. The matrix, or modified versions, would be adaptable to a variety of commissioning arrangements

Table 2.5 Possible framework for service-level agreement for school nursing services (source: DOH, 1994)

Health of the nation targets	Professional involvement	Opportunities for health-promoting activities
To reduce the rate for accidents among children aged under 15 by at least (33%) for women by the year 2005	Teacher	In the classroom, linked with National Curriculum subjects
	School nurse	Group work with parents
	Health promotion officer	Talks given by emergency services and others at school assemblies
	Police	Provision of school cycling lessons
		Arrangements with local shops for a reduction in the cost of safety equipment
To reduce the percentages of men and women aged 16–64 who are obese by at least 25% for men and at least 33% for women by the year 2005	Teacher (PE teacher)	Time built into the timetable for physical activity
	School nurse	Structured games and activities at play-time
	Health promotion officer	After schools clubs
	Doctors	Reduced rates for admission to local sports centre
	Local sports centre	School projects, e.g. a Fun Run
	Dietician	Healthy nutrition included in the National Curriculum

between providers and purchasers such as PCGs, PCTs, commissioning pilots or health and social services Boards with different populations, deprivation weightings and priorities. Most importantly in the context of this chapter, it is a vehicle for facilitating public health practice across all five dimensions identified by Holman (1992), with a reorientation away from 'how many?' towards 'good practice based on identified need'.

In the effort to promote public health practice, a major strategic goal must be to achieve effective integration of primary care and public health. The Public Health Alliance (PHA) (PHA, 1998) has developed a public health model of primary care where primary care is conceived as more than medical care, health determinants are acknowledged as environmental, biological, social and lifestyle-related, communities are active in addressing health issues and equity, participation and collaboration are the drivers for the delivery of primary care. In a two-year study, the PHA found that factors such as over-emphasis on 'individuals' prevented the two sectors from overlapping, whereas encouragement of participation by lay people and community groups drew the two sectors together.

A positive recent development is the top priority assigned to 'addressing health inequalities' as the first function of a PCG (DOH England, 2000a). It is also significant that PCTs are mandated to employ a 'public health member' on their executive committees (DOH England, 2000c). Furthermore, of the maximum membership of 15 on the PCT Executive Committee, 'professional representation' must include a number of medical practitioners (not exceeding seven) and a number of nurses (not exceeding seven). If the medical and nursing representation proves to be balanced, this could be an unprecedented opportunity for community nurses to drive forward a truly public health-orientated primary care agenda.

ORGANIZATIONAL MEASURES TO STRENGTHEN THE NURSING CONTRIBUTION TO PUBLIC HEALTH

Four models have been suggested for accommodating public health practice in community nursing (Mason, 1995; Hoskins, 2000).

The creation of specialist health visitors in public health, who work alongside their caseload-holding colleagues

An early, well-documented example of this model was the Strelley Nursing Development Unit (SNDU) in Nottingham (SNDU, 1993; Jackson, 1994) where a full-time post was assigned for public health work. The health visitor completed a community health profile and identified accident prevention as a target area for health improvement. Collaboration with the local community and organizations such as education, social services, housing, environmental health, the voluntary sector and the health service produced a low-cost home safety equipment system, basic first aid courses, more public telephones and a welfare rights advice session one day per week at the local library. Follow-up projects, at the request of local women, included a baby drop-in, which 'is more like a group than a clinic', and a women's aid advice service launched in response to the known incidence of domestic violence. Since 'Strelley', many community development projects have been initiated successfully by community nurses with a specialist public health remit (see, for example, Lazenbatt (1997) for a directory of 'targeting health and social need' projects). A significant benefit is that specialist public health community nurses can liaise closely with caseload-holding colleagues to assess health and social needs. Specialist public health nurses in Glasgow are offering community development training to their local community colleagues, and an up-to-date database of current community nurse public health activity has been developed (Greater Glasgow Primary Care NHS Trust, 2000).

Separation of the public health function from the generic role of the community nurse or health visitor: different employers and different agendas

This has been advocated by Barker (1993) who envisaged (a) practice health visitors focusing on generic family and child health promotion and prevention and (b) 'all community' health visitors employed by FHSAs or public health directorates. As Hoskins (2000) indicates, this would have the advantage that health visitors could select the type of work with which they feel most comfortable. In addition, if public health visitors were part of public health directorates, this could facilitate inter-professional and inter-sectoral working for public health. Furthermore, the tension for health visitors between primary care and public health would be averted: the public health function would be aligned with public health departments while primary care oriented work would 'sit' with general practice/ PCGs. On the other hand, questions remain about how generic health visitors would cope with larger caseloads as some of the health visiting resource is siphoned off into community public health.

A register of public health practitioners

Further separation of the role of the public health nurse would be achieved in a new scenario where all public health practitioners, from different disciplines, would be drawn together with a 'common identity' (Watkins, 1992). A joint register of public health practitioners could be established. Current trends indicate a move in this direction, for example, the UK Public Health Association* (UKPHA) has composite membership from a wide range of voluntary and statutory sectors, organizations and individuals. Launched in 1999, its mission is

> . . . to act as a unifying and powerful force to promote the public's health and wellbeing. The UKPHA supports everyone in public health,

*UK Public Health Association, 58 Langdale Road, Manchester M4 5PN (tel: 0870 0101932; email: report@ukpha.org.uk).

whether working professionally or in a voluntary capacity. It works in partnership with other organisations in the UK and internationally to create a healthy, sustainable and equitable society.

Similarly, the recently established Institute of Public Health in Ireland (IPHI) is an open, multi-sectoral organization aiming 'to improve health in Ireland, by working to combat health inequalities and influence public policies in favour of health' (IPHI, 2000).

Issues around professional registration as public health practitioner are increasingly being confronted. For example, medical public health consultants follow a 13–14-year pathway, including specified clinical experiences and an academic thesis to MPhil level. Other professions tend to have less-established routes, yet many – and perhaps especially epidemiologists – argue that there must be a recognized public health career pathway and professional status. Healthwork UK* has recently been commissioned by the Department of Health England to consult widely on these issues, across the UK and with a range of professionals.

Ad hoc integration of the public health function within generic community nursing/health visiting

This is probably the most common way that public health is practised in community nursing today. Many health visitors, for example, argue that their family support role facilitates the assessment of family and community health needs, and encourages tailored projects, groupwork, health promotion and links with voluntary sector bodies such as NewPin, Lifestart or Homestart. Similarly, school nurses could argue that their expanding role in developing school health profiles and healthy school policies in partnership with education, is an excellent example of effective integration of public health into professional school nursing. Moreover, public health as categorized by Holman (1992) is incorporated into the generic work of all community nurses; it is important not to demean secondary and tertiary prevention – cost-effective screening, immunization, diabetic foot care, etc. and health education – amidst the apparent growth in community- and population-focused public health. It appears that the English Department of Health is promoting this fourth model. *Saving Lives: Our Healthier Nation* (DOH England, 1999a) advocates for health visitors, school nurses and midwives, a range of functions that cover public health both as population-centred and also public health as individualized support and advice.

Interestingly, the population-centred and client-centred models of public health are used simultaneously in many countries in Europe and the comparative benefits and costs of each are constantly under review. No one model has emerged as singularly effective.

*The Health Care National Training Organisation, 344–345 Gray's Inn Road, London WC1 8PB (tel: 020 7692 5550; email: office@healthwork.co.uk).

In Europe as a whole, further debate surrounds the extent to which specialization is desirable. The UK is possibly at the extreme end of the spectrum in favour of having a wide range of specialisms. Arguably, this creates fragmentation and potential duplication. However, at the other end of the spectrum, problems have been identified with the unified public health nurse role in the Republic of Ireland, where there is a risk that health promotion may be subsumed by the more immediate demands of curative care (Government of Ireland, 1994). The trend in that country appears to be towards greater specialization.

The WHO is currently promoting the concept of the family nurse: a generic, multi-skilled practitioner who, along with the family physician, would be at the centre of primary health care services. Some European Member States already have these categories of worker, while many do not. *Health 21* (WHO, 1988) views the family nurse as having a unified health promoting, preventive and caregiving function, focusing on families and individuals and substituting for the family physician when the identified needs are more relevant to nursing expertise. The extent to which the family health nurse model will be adopted in the UK remains to seen. It would seem unwise to fragment the range of community nurse specialisms still further by adding another category; however there may be potential for coalescing existing health visiting, midwifery and district nursing skills, for example, to produce a more generic, family-orientated nurse. It is unclear how this would complement the role of the nurse practitioner. The family health nurse role is presently being piloted in Scotland.

PROFESSIONAL MEASURES TO STRENGTHEN THE NURSING CONTRIBUTION TO PUBLIC HEALTH

Professional measures for enhancement of the public health role in community nursing centre on education, leadership and quality standards and governance. It has been demonstrated that community nurses feel well-prepared to carry out health education and primary, secondary and tertiary prevention, but inadequately educated for community-focused public health, including planning, developing, implementing and evaluating public health projects (Poulton *et al.*, 2000). This suggests that the public health component of pre- and post-registration courses should be strengthened. There is a strong argument that public health modules and courses should be not only multi-professional but multi-agency, and that complementary methods of delivering public health education, for example by distance learning and/or the internet, should be explored.

Similarly, leadership for public health in nursing needs to be enhanced to drive forward the public health agenda. The Scotland review of nursing and public health (Scottish Executive, 2000) suggests that this is needed at all levels, but in a way that does not add to hierarchies. With respect to quality standards and governance, the Scottish consultation indicated that, since much of the creative public health improvement work by nurses occurs on the margins of 'normal' activity, it is difficult to regulate in terms of quality.

Meaningful standards therefore need to be developed at all levels, along with professional and organizational accountability for delivering on the public heath agenda. It follows that the evidence base for public health work needs to be expanded and used as the basis for practice.

Conclusion

This chapter began by asking the question 'Can the public health agenda really be a part of community nursing?' It has been argued that 'public health' encompasses a range of activities, including health protection, prevention, health education, healthy public policy and community empowerment. All community nursing specialisms incorporate these dimensions of public health into their work to a greater or lesser extent and in this sense the public health agenda is part of community nursing. However, there is generally a concentration on prevention and health promotion with a weaker focus on community empowerment and healthy public policy. For reasons that have been explored, it appears that community nursing in the UK is primarily client- and family-centred rather than population-centred.

If we take a more global view of public health presented for example in the *Ottawa Charter* (WHO, 1986), it is apparent that community nursing alone can have only a limited influence, for example, on reorientation of health service priorities and environmental policy. The public health agenda in this sense may form part of the underpinning ethos of community nursing aligning easily, for instance, with the principles of health visiting. However, when the public health agenda is defined as organized social and political effort for health improvement, it may be more meaningful to ask how community nursing can *contribute* to that agenda. It has been suggested here that community nurses have a vital contribution to make: as health workers who 'know' local culture and have the trust of local people, community nurses are in a key position to assess the kinds of social, environmental and health measures that are needed for health improvement. An important and achievable challenge for community nursing would be to mobilize this knowledge, translating it into action by influencing PCTs and collaborating with organizations such as the UKPHA and other bodies who can harness the collective professional and voluntary expertise to effectively lobby for social and political change for health.

References

Acheson, R. (1988) *Public health in England — the report of the committee of inquiry into the future development of the public health function. Cm289.* London: HMSO.

Barker, W. (1993) Patch and practice: specialist roles for health visitors. *Health Visitor*, 66: 200–3.

Baum, F., Traynor, M. and Brice, G. (1992) Healthy cities: the Noarlunga experience. In: Gardner, H. (ed.) *Health policy development, implementation and evaluation in Australia.* Melbourne: Churchill Livingstone.

Chief Nursing Officers Report. (1998) *The nursing and midwifery contribution to the public health agenda in the European Union — report and recommendations of the United Kingdom European Union Presidency Chief Nursing Officers' meeting 13/14 May 1998.*

CETHV. (1977) *An investigation into the principles of health visiting.* London: CETHV.

CPHVA/QNI/RCN. (2000) *School nursing within the public health agenda. A Strategy for Practice.* London: McMillan-Scott.

CPHVA. (1999) *Joined up working: community development in primary health care.* London: CPHVA.

DHSSPS. (2000) *Investing for health. A consultation document.* DHSSPS.

Department of Health England. (1994) *Negotiating school health services.* London: DOH.

Department of Heath England. (1997) *The new NHS: modern, dependable.* London: DOH.

Department of Health England. (1999a) *Saving lives: our healthier nation.* London: DOH.

Department of Health England. (2000a) *Primary care Trusts.* London: DOH (http://www.doh.gov.uk/pricare/pcts.htm).

Department of Health England. (2000b) *The NHS plan. A plan for investment. A plan for reform.* London: DOH.

Department of Health England. (2000c) National Health Service Act 1977. *The primary care Trust executive committees (membership) (no. 2) directions 2000.* London: DOH.

Department of Health Scotland. (1998) *Working together for a healthier Scotland.* Edinburgh: DOH.

Department of Health Wales. (1998) *Better health, better Wales.* Cardiff: The Stationery Office.

Government of Ireland. (1994) *A service without walls — an analysis of public health nursing.* Dublin: The Stationery Office.

Greater Glasgow Primary Care NHS Trust. (2000) *Health visitor review: the public health contribution of health visitors.* Glasgow: Greater Glasgow Primary Care NHS Trust.

Holman, J. (1992) Something old, something new: perspectives on five 'new' public health movements. *Health Promotion Journal of Australia,* 2: 4–11.

Hoskins, R. (2000) Public health: a new nursing role for community practitioners. *British Journal of Community Nursing,* 2000 5: 246–53.

Institute of Medicine. (1988) *The future of public health.* Washington: National Academy Press.

Institute of Public Health in Ireland. (IPHI) (2000) *The Institute of Public Health in Ireland. Strategic plan 2000–2003.* Dublin: IPHI.

Jackson, C. (1994) Strelley: teamworking for health. *Health Visitor,* 67: 28–9.

Lazenbatt, A. (1997) *Targeting health and social need. The contribution of nurses, midwives and health visitors — directory of survey respondents.* Belfast: DHSSPS.

Macdonald, J. (1992) *Primary health care: medicine in its place.* London: Earthscan.

Mason, C. (1995) Towards public health nursing. In: Sines, D. (ed.) *Community health care nursing.* Oxford: Blackwell.

Poulton, B., Mason, C., McKenna, H., Lynch, C. and Keeney, S. (2000) *The contribution of nurses, midwives and health visitors to the public health agenda in Northern Ireland.* Belfast: DHSSPS.

Public Health Alliance. (1998) *A public health model of primary care — from concept to reality.* Birmingham: Public Health Alliance.

Royal College of Nursing. (1994) *Public health: nursing rises to the challenge.* London: RCN.

Sandhu, G. (1996) Genesis of primary health care. In: *Rural primary health care: distance education course CRH1012.* Victoria: Monash University.

Southern Health and Social Services Board. (1997) *Primary care strategy.* Armagh: Southern Health and Social Services Board Northern Ireland.

Scottish Executive. (2000) *Review of the nurses contribution to improving the public's health. Consultation on the main findings 26 June — 27 August 2000.* Scotland: Scottish Executive.

Strelley Nursing Development Unit. (1993) *The public health post at Strelley: an interim report.* Nottingham, Strelley NDU.

Twinn, S. and Cowley, S. (1992) *The principles of health visiting. A re-examination.* London: HVA.

Watkins, S.J. (1992) A route from two roots. *Health Visitor*, 65: 111.

World Health Organization. (1948) Constitution. Geneva: WHO.

World Health Organization. (1986) *Ottawa Charter for health promotion.* Geneva: WHO.

World Health Organization. (1998) *Health 21 — health for all in the 21st century.* Copenhagen: WHO.

World Health Organization. (2000) *Munich declaration. Nurses and midwives: a force for health.* Copenhagan: WHO EUR/00/50193096/6.

3 Assessing health needs: putting policy into practice

Sandy Tinson and Kath Hutchinson

Introduction

A sensible starting point for any practitioner embarking upon an assessment of health need is a clear understanding of the two key terms 'health' and 'need'. Once their meanings are established practitioners should then have a clearer notion of what should be assessed and how this is best achieved. However, this apparently logical approach is not as easy as it may at first appear, as the literature reveals little consensus on the meaning of either 'health' or 'need' and even less in defining the scope of 'assessment' (Kilduff *et al.*, 1998). This is remarkable, not least because from its inception in 1948, the National Health Service (NHS) has aspired to be a needs-led service. Health needs assessment has been promoted by successive governments as a mechanism which can identify and prioritize areas for development and improve the health and health care of local populations. However, the context and rationale for health needs assessment has changed over time according to the changing political and economic agenda.

The NHS was introduced by the Labour government in 1948, albeit with a great deal of opposition from both Conservative politicians and many within the medical profession, to provide a service which met the health needs of the whole population. Economic and social status would no longer be the determinants of health, and health care would be free and accessible to all. Beveridge, who was regarded as the founder of the NHS, believed that once the health needs of the population had been met by this new service, the costs would diminish accordingly. As we are all too aware, this was certainly not the reality. Changes in demographic trends, advances in technology and increasing expectations of consumers, all combined to increase the cost of the NHS. Little more than 30 years later, the NHS was seen by the Conservative government of the day, not as a benevolent provider of health care, but as a wasteful consumer of public money with little regard for the quality or efficiency of its service provision. This hypothesis set in motion the changes of the next 20 years which sought to create a more business-like health service, that would be better able to meet the changing health demands of the future.

Therefore, within this context, assessing the health needs of a local population was seen as the key component in effective targeting of health care services and a more appropriate use of health resources (DOH, 1989).

However, despite the high priority given to health needs assessment and targeting of resources throughout the 1980s and 1990s there is still evidence to suggest a widening gap in the health status of certain groups within the population (DOH, 1998). The poor and disadvantaged, whose health needs are clearly not being addressed within current health care provision, still represent a large section of the population.

Over half a century has passed since the inception of the NHS and, predictably, health needs assessment is still high on the political agenda. The New Labour government has committed itself to ensuring access to treatment according to 'need and need alone' (DOH, 1997). This chapter will discuss the impact of the most recent health care policy on health needs assessment. It will clarify the definition of health need within the context of the 'New NHS' and will suggest the most effective way community nurses can work in collaboration with other professionals and agencies to address health needs within the current economic and political agenda. Finally, a case study is used to illustrate a systematic approach to health needs assessment within the current health economy.

Health needs assessment: a new agenda for action?

From the time the new Labour government came into power in May 1997, there has been a rapid programme of structural and policy reforms that has changed the value base and direction of national health policy. However, the shift to a more community-focused form of health care is not new as this process had already begun with the previous Conservative government. The White Paper, *Promoting Better Health* (DOH, 1987), encouraged primary health care teams to be more responsive to identified need and to set clear priorities for care which emphasized the contribution of health promotion and disease prevention. The overall aim of the subsequent NHS Act (DOH, 1990) was to provide efficient and effective health care for individuals and communities alike, based on need. The introduction of the general practitioner (GP) contract and subsequent developments and innovations in GP fundholding established the pivotal role of general practice and primary care in providing a wide range of health care services which met the specific health needs of individual practice populations.

The White Paper, *The New NHS: Modern and Dependable* (DOH, 1997) introduced the concept of a 'third way' for health and social reform. It also stressed the importance of needs assessment to the planning and provision of health care, although it marked the end of the internal market. This was a model that required greater public participation and social responsibility from the community. It was a health care system based on 'partnership and driven by performance' and once again the assessment of health and social need became an integral part of the Government's reforms and initiatives. A selection of some of the most recent policy initiatives arising from these reforms is discussed below and clearly indicates the significance of health need assessment to their implementation.

PRIMARY CARE GROUPS

The most notable development for primary health care was that local doctors and nurses should work together in Primary Care Groups (PCGs) to plan, purchase and commission health and social care on the basis of health need. The White Paper (DOH, 1997) clearly acknowledged that community nurses and doctors were best-placed to identify patient need and to ensure that health care provision was responsive to meet those needs. Therefore, PCGs offer local nurses and doctors 'the opportunity to deploy resources and savings to strengthen local services and ensure that patterns of care best reflect their patients' needs' (DOH, 1997).

The four-tier system of PCGs is intended to make health services more public health-focused and health needs assessment is seen as integral to the process by which primary care responds to local and national priorities in the promotion of effective and equitable care (Jordan *et al.*, 1998).

HEALTH IMPROVEMENT PROGRAMMES

Each Health Authority has been given the task of developing local Health Improvement Programmes (HImPs). It is intended that these will focus upon the determinants of health and will improve the health of the local population through partnership with the non-health sector. PCGs are required to contribute to these HImPs in collaboration with NHS Trusts, local authorities, other primary care professionals, the public and other partner organizations. The HImPs are the local strategies for improving health and health care and will identify the way national targets are addressed within each Health Authority. The HImPs will identify:

- The health needs of the local population and how they are to be met by the NHS and its partner organizations.
- The healthcare requirements of the local population and how they are to be met by local services.
- The range, location and investment required in local health services to meet the needs of local people.
- The initial HImPs will cover a three-year period and will be updated progressively and reviewed each year. The HImPs are intended to be the driving force behind future health care policy and practice.

HEALTH ACTION ZONES

The Government has identified funds to support a number of health action zones in areas of particular need. These will mostly be in urban areas with significant, identified deprivation where specific action is required. Applications for funding will be dependent on all local agencies working together. This will typically include health, social services, industry, commerce and the community itself, all working together to fund and support local initiatives.

SAVING LIVES

Saving Lives: Our Healthier Nation (DOH, 1999a) is an action plan to tackle poor health and health inequality. It builds on the initial *The Health of the Nation* strategy (DOH, 1992) and sets out targets for health in priority areas (cancer, coronary heart disease and stroke, accidents and mental illness) and, at last, acknowledges the impact of social, economic and environmental factors upon the health of individuals and communities. The original document (DOH, 1992) could never bring about all the required improvements without commitment from the other government departments (Fatchett, 1998). Consequently, in line with this recent policy, the Government introduced a range of initiatives on education, welfare to work, housing, neighbourhood, transport and the environment 'to improve health' (DOH, 1998). HImPs also address the national and local health targets contained within the document and health needs assessment will be a key component in achieving changes in the mortality and morbidity of the identified target areas. It is particularly significant that local authorities must be seen to be working in partnership with the NHS to achieve these changes.

SUPPORTING FAMILIES

The consultation document, *Supporting Families,* was published in November 1998 (Home Office, 1998a) and set out the Government's proposals for a package of practical measures to increase the support available to families. Its intention is that existing services and structures should be extended and strengthened to provide more effective support for families. The document looks at five key areas:

- Better services and support to parents.
- Better financial support to families.
- Helping families balance work and home.
- Strengthening marriage.
- Better support for serious family problems.

Following publication of *Supporting Families* (Home Office, 1998a) there have been various initiatives and developments intended to push this work forward. They have included the Sure Start programme, Parentline and the Innovation Fund for health visiting and school nursing, in addition to other developments within education, employment and the youth justice system.

SURE START

The Sure Start Initiative is described in the *Supporting Families* (Home Office, 1998a) document and will contribute to the Government's strategy to reduce inequalities. The intention of Sure Start is to build on and add value to local services for families. The aim is to improve services for families within a designated area through the provision of a more co-ordinated approach to the planning and delivery of health and social care for parents and carers. Where families are in great need Sure Start will provide further support and advice on parenting, primary health care, early learning, play opportunities and child care. This will promote physical, intellectual, social and emotional development in children so that they are better prepared to learn at school. Sure Start schemes can also involve parents in supporting literacy, numeracy and life skills training which can improve future employment prospects (Home Office, 1998). In line with the White Paper (DOH, 1997) it will build on existing local services and promote partnership working between voluntary and statutory agencies. Local businesses, parents, community volunteers, primary health care teams, education and other child care professionals within the community will provide an integrated service that will concentrate resources on those in greatest need and promote social change by addressing the deficiencies associated with low socio-economic status (Whitehead, 1992).

Defining health needs

Health needs assessment is a problematic concept because the 'assessors' usually view health needs from their own perspective. The economist, epidemiologist, public health physician and community nurse will all offer their own bias to the assessment process. This is not necessarily a problem but practitioners should always be aware of the potential for bias in their assessment process and subsequent analysis.

The sociologist's view, and one that still remains the cornerstone of health need assessment is clearly illustrated by Bradshaw's Taxonomy of Need (Bradshaw, 1972). His account of *normative* need, *felt* need, *expressed* need and *comparative* need was discussed in detail by Tinson (1995). This account remains a valid framework for the assessment process but it does not always provide the detailed information required by those who are actively involved in setting priorities and planning and commissioning future health care provision (Stevens and Raftery, 1997).

There is a variety of sources of information currently being utilized in the assessment of health needs. The most familiar of these are the measures of morbidity and mortality. Social need is more usually addressed by measurement of a population's deprivation, e.g. the Jarman score (Jarman, 1983). All of these measures provide valuable information about a population's unmet needs. However, these measures do not necessarily inform planners of the *specific* need for health care (Stevens and Gabbay, 1991), particularly within a local population.

It may be helpful at this point to discuss the subtle difference between the need for *health* and the need for *health care*.

Health needs incorporate the wider influences upon health, such as housing, education, behaviour, socio-economic status and genetic disposition.

Health care needs are those that can benefit from the provision of health care. These can incorporate all forms of health care, such as health education, disease prevention and rehabilitation, as well as treatment.

Within the current context of health care provision, Stevens and Raftery (1997) have defined health need as 'the population's ability to benefit from health care'. Their definition recognizes that:

- Resources should be utilized according to need.
- Resources are finite.

This definition, although in contrast with the broader public health definition of health needs demonstrated in *Saving Lives* (DOH, 1998a), does acknowledge the significance of resources being available to meet these needs. Within this context it is helpful to differentiate health need in terms of 'need', 'demand' and 'supply'.

Need, demand and supply

A *health need* can be defined as that which, if met, will result in an improvement in people's health. This need may vary over time and is subject to a variety of influences. These influences can include cultural and ethical determinants, such as the need for interpreters or multilingual health education literature in some communities.

It can also be influenced by research or the current political agenda. For example, Sure Start with its emphasis on children's health and education needs may determine the health needs assessment agenda within specific areas of deprivation.

It is important to recognize that the 'ability to benefit' from health care may not be the same for all members of the population. For example, if screening clinics are only available in GP surgeries there may be a significant number of the population who would find this type of provision unacceptable for a variety of cultural or social reasons.

It is also worth noting that a benefit is not always measured in terms of clinical outcome but could refer to quality of the health care. This could be judged by the level of reassurance a patient gains from an interaction with a health professional. How often is patient satisfaction seen as a viable measure of health care?

The complexity of changing health need is represented by the following example. The need for daily insulin injections from the district nurse has reduced for two reasons. First, because of improved technology and, second, because patients have taken over the role originally thought to belong to the nurse alone.

Demand is what people ask for, are willing to pay for or might wish to use in a system of free care. Demand can also be dependent upon many variables. It could arise from media interest, individuals' own educational and cultural influences, or practitioners' own bias and belief. For example, if a community nurse has benefited from acupuncture or is a registered acupuncturist, patients' demand for this type of intervention may be increased.

Demand can be measured in a variety of ways. Currently, the most significant and contentious measure is waiting lists. However, the measure may show a regional or geographical difference in demand, which in the case of waiting lists may have more to do with individual practitioners' referral patterns or the level and type of regional health care provision, rather than actual patient need.

Supply is the health care actually provided. This, too, can be shaped by a variety of influences. These can range from the current political agenda or local public pressure, to the availability of resources. It can also be determined through historical patterns of care or even inertia and an inability to change. The age-old issue of 'social baths' may be a case in point here. District nurses are still requested to provide baths which address a social rather than a health need.

Need, demand and supply are interdependent (Figure 3.1). Any assessment of need will require an assessment of the relationship between all three: need, demand and supply. The objective is to establish how the three can be made more congruent. In other words, how need, demand and supply can be more closely related (Figure 3.2).

Most of the health service information currently available relates to supply, for example utilization rates; and demand, for example patient satisfaction surveys. There seems to be very little information about need. Future health care commissioners should strive to bring together need, supply and demand. In other words identify:

- What people ask for.
- What they will benefit from.
- What they can be supplied (Johnstone, 1999).

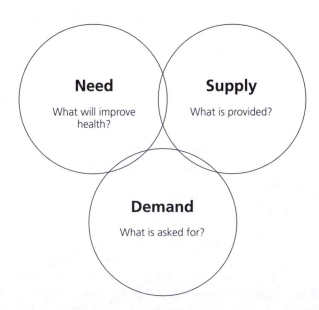

Figure 3.1 The three elements of health needs assessment: need, supply and demand

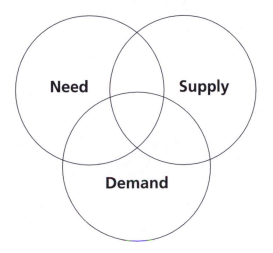

Figure 3.2 The relationship between need, supply and demand

EXAMPLES FROM PRACTICE

The following three examples of health care have been chosen to illustrate the interaction between need, demand and supply.

Child health surveillance

Need

The Hall report (Hall, 1996) has shown that there is no longer a need for the same level of routine child developmental surveillance and home visiting by health visitors. The introduction of parent-held records, self-assessment questionnaires and targeted home visits have reduced the need for such interventions.

Demand

Parents in some areas may demand the same high number of home visits from the health visitor. This may be due to their own social and educational characteristics, the established visiting pattern of the health visitor or the rural characteristic of the community which requires that the health visitor has to visit them at home rather than them coming to the clinic.

Supply

This reflects the actual provision of child health surveillance in the home by the health visitor. This may be influenced by a variety of factors. These could include the health visitor's personal preference, historical patterns of visiting or characteristics of the population. It may also reflect the particular infrastructure that exists within that area, for example, poor transport systems or a small number of households with a telephone.

Leg ulcer care

Need

Research (Moffatt and Dolman, 1995) has shown the benefits of the correct assessment, diagnosis and treatment of leg ulcers. This has resulted in an increase in the use of four-layer bandaging for venous leg ulcers. This, combined with a good diet, increases the outcome of treatment. It also reduces the need for the district nurse to visit for daily dressings, as was sometimes the case before this treatment. These bandages must be obtained on prescription.

Demand

Patients may not be aware of these benefits and sometimes find it hard to understand that a bandage left for several days will be just as effective, if not more effective, than daily dressings. Leg ulcers rarely attract national media interest and therefore the chance of a patient asking for this type of intervention is rare. It is up to the diligence and knowledge base of the district nurse to use evidence-based practice and employ this form of effective treatment.

Supply

These bandages are expensive and this may have limited their use in practice. They will have been viewed as a cost pressure for the general practice and therefore the nurse may have been told that this type of treatment was not an option because of the economic burden. The introduction of nurse prescribing may affect prescribing patterns, although the cost pressure still remains and may remain an influence on the supply. It has been shown that expenditure on four-layer bandaging is far less than the cost of daily dressings over a long period of time (Kings Fund, 1998); therefore, through the introduction of evidence-based practice, the measure of supply may change over time.

Stevens and Gabbay (1991) believe that the ideal scenario would bring the three elements closer together, so that everything that is supplied is both needed and recognized as such by everyone. The outcome would be that, over time, the NHS would become more effective and efficient. This perspective would be extremely worthwhile when undertaking any needs assessment process within the community, as it clarifies the issues and identifies the need for further action in the future.

What does health needs assessment mean for community nurses?

Health needs assessment enables practitioners to respond to the community's health needs rather than reacting to its demands. It enables community nurses to work collaboratively with others to:

- Describe patterns of disease and deprivation in local populations and compare them with regional variations and the national perspective. This will identify the extent of need.
- Learn more about the needs and priorities of the local population.
- Identify inequalities in health and access to services.
- Identify local need through consultation with users and other professionals and find out more about the implications for users and the health care service.
- Highlight areas of unmet need and establish ways to address those needs.
- Determine priorities for action and how these can best be addressed within the resources available.
- Identify those services where people can benefit from health care and/or from social or environmental change.
- Enable health resources to be used in the most efficient way to benefit and improve the health of the population.
- Balance clinical, ethical and economic considerations.
- Influence policy, inter-agency collaboration and research priorities.

In order to achieve this a variety of approaches and methods is required.

Different perspectives of needs assessment

THE MEDICAL MODEL OF NEEDS ASSESSMENT

The medical model measures need in terms of the occurrence of specific diseases or health-related states within communities (Williams and Wright, 1998). It does not necessarily consider groups of people within a community but looks more at the pattern of disease. Therefore, it represents the *epidemiological* approach to health needs assessment. This approach asks:

- *Who* are the affected people?
- *Where* are they and what is the *prevalence* and *incidence* of the disease/ condition?
- *When* do they get the disease?

Although the measures of the incidence and prevalence of disease do not necessarily equate with need, Williams and Wright (1998) believe they are important in describing the burden of the disease within the community. For example:

- The incidence and prevalence of meningococcal C in a community may be very significant. It would identify a need for specific immunization and health education programmes, particularly within a university town or city which has a high proportion of young adults at high risk.
- The prevalence of asthma within a specific community would be significant, as the long term treatment of this type of condition would have an impact on economic and resource distribution over time.

Measures used in an epidemiological assessment could include:

- Standardized mortality ratio (SMR).
- Admission rates.
- Operation rates.
- Discharge rates.
- Length of stay in hospital.
- Townsend or Jarman score (deprivation according to ward).
- Morbidity data.
- Mortality data.
- Age/Sex ratio.

THE SOCIAL MODEL OF NEEDS ASSESSMENT

Saving Lives (DOH, 1999a) clearly identifies a public health agenda that recognizes that the social determinants of health which include housing, education, socio-economic status, transport and employment all have an impact upon health need. The Acheson Report (DOH, 1998) offered a more uncompromising analysis of health inequality and showed that the distribution and degree of inequality in economic terms has a direct impact upon health. It stated that without a shift in resources to the less well-off there will be little reduction in health inequality in the foreseeable future.

The social model acknowledges the impact of social determinants upon health and their influence on the uptake and access to health care. Individuals and communities can only *benefit* from health care if they find it both acceptable and accessible. Language and culture, transport and education can all have an effect on the uptake and utilization of health care or the identified 'demand'. Housing can also have a direct impact on disease patterns. Poor housing can increase the incidence of respiratory disease, accidents, mental illness and poor nutrition.

Measurements of social need could include:

- Jarman deprivation score.
- Townsend score.
- Un/employment.
- Housing type.
- Ethnicity.
- Socio-economic status.
- Disability.
- Age.
- Crime.
- Numbers per household.
- Transport systems.
- Car ownership.
- One-parent families.

THE ECONOMIC MODEL OF HEALTH NEEDS ASSESSMENT

This chapter has already given a brief overview of the changing focus of health needs assessment within the NHS. It has described how health needs assessment has sought to serve several different political purposes over the years. The economic model was particularly prevalent during the Thatcher government and shaped the development of the internal market. More recently, it has become clear that if health needs assessment is to have any value in the future, health care arising from it should not only be clinically and/or socially effective but also cost-effective. The economic model of health needs assessment will always want to consider current service provision; any shortfall between need, demand and supply will affect the overall effectiveness of the intervention. The economist will always make the assumption that needs will always outstrip the resources available and therefore consideration of the effectiveness of an intervention will assist in the consideration of the relative priority of different needs.

Need assessments that fail to acknowledge resource limitations can be of restricted use when commissioning health care. There is always a danger of this when health professionals undertake individual needs assessment. The care programme approach (CPA) in mental health is a good example of this. In this instance, assessment of patient need focuses on what is best for individual patients within their own environments. This approach, although considered to be the best solution, may put great pressure on restricted budgets. It may also disadvantage those client groups with a weak advocacy structure who require a more political approach to identifying their groups' needs. However, population needs assessments can also fail to recognize resource implications and there is always a danger that recommendations based on lobbying will result in extreme and inappropriate demands on resources (Stevens and Raftery, 1997).

Measurements used in an economic model of needs assessment could include:

- Evidence-based practice, e.g. the Cochrane database.
- Research.
- NHS performance indicators.
- Cost per unit of care/outcome.
- Delayed discharge.
- Readmission rates
- Population need.
- Quality adjusted life year (QALY).

Which approach is best?

Different approaches to health needs assessment are employed according to their intended purpose and context. Stevens and Raftery (1997) have identified the following questions to assist in determining the approaches:

- *Is the principal concern with health or social services?* Compared to health, social service need may not always be associated with effectiveness. How can new housing or more education be shown to directly contribute to improved health? The current agenda however, does at least acknowledge the contribution of both perspectives.
- *Is the needs assessment about populations or individuals?* Health care is usually commissioned on the basis of the identified needs of the aggregate population. Individual need should not be forgotten, as minority groups, such as those with a learning disability, should have their specific needs considered alongside that of the wider population.
- *Is there a clear context of allocating scarce resources?* Health care has to work within an implicit resource framework. Although population health care needs assessment must acknowledge resource issues it should not be driven by this approach alone.
- *Is the needs assessment about priority setting or is it about advocacy for a single group or individual?* Policy directives which focus on specific agendas, may distort resource utilization. The allocation of resources is dependent upon meeting the needs and priorities identified within specific initiatives or policies.
- *Is the needs assessment exploratory or definitive?* Some approaches to health needs assessment actually highlight previously undefined health need. This may happen when specific groups are surveyed, for example, teenage alcohol abusers. If this comes to light it is necessary to ask to what extent do these comply with the health care agenda?
- *Is the determination of the most important needs expert-led or participatory?* Epidemiology provides the expert approach to needs assessment. It is, as far as possible, an objective assessment of need. Stevens and Raftery (1997) believe that the expert approach to priority setting is more viable the further away it is from the clinical decision making. However these authors also acknowledge that the clinician is also open to the patient view and the two should be reconciled in some way. The qualitative approach to health needs assessment should be as rigorous as the epidemiological.

These questions clearly demonstrate that different approaches can be both valid and complementary within health needs assessment. However, although health needs assessment represents an amalgam of epidemiology, economics and values, it has to be turned into a practical tool. Community nurses need to be aware that there are some adverse effects to this.

IT IS NOT ALWAYS A LOGICAL PROCESS

Stevens and Gillam (1998) believe that it is unhelpful to see health needs assessment as a single document, which is 'a culmination of a series of easily defined steps'. Historically, community nurses have often viewed the community profile as the only health needs assessment tool for the community. In fact, it should be a combination of methods which achieves some agreement between planners, managers and practitioners in setting priorities.

IT IS NOT THE PRESERVE OF THE PUBLIC HEALTH SPECIALIST

It does not need highly developed technical skills. Community nurses, through health profiling already have the necessary skills to contribute to the wider health needs assessment agenda. They have local knowledge and work at many levels with many agencies but they must ensure these skills are recognized and appreciated within PCGs and developing PCTs (Hipkin *et al.*, 1999).

It is clear that any future health needs assessment should involve a wide range of information sources, which not only involve professionals and the voluntary sector but also service users, their families and carers.

User participation in health needs assessment

In the past, consultation with users has been largely a rhetorical concept. The obligation of health care planners to consult with current users and the public in general has been clearly stated (DOH, 1997). Although there may have been an increase in public involvement in recent years the quality of this process has been questionable (Jordan *et al.*, 1998). Surveys and consultation with local user groups have remained the most frequently adopted approaches. This has remained a largely passive exercise for the users and they have frequently been asked for their views with little knowledge of the issues or opportunity to develop their opinions and thoughts.

The necessity for health care to respond to specific local needs has made it essential to involve users in decisions about health care. It is all too easy for health practitioners to assume that they 'know the needs of their community'. The majority of the community does not come into contact with the health care professionals and most illnesses do not come into contact with the health care system. Contact with health care professionals is only one expression of demand. It is important to remember this, as it is especially significant if inequalities of health are to be addressed. However, there is a danger that those members of the public who are most able to register their demands or needs do so at the expense of the less articulate (Percy-Smith and Sanderson, 1992) and it is imperative that minority groups are involved in this consultation process.

The following methods of public consultation have been identified by Jordan *et al.* (1998):

- *Citizens' juries*: participants are selected as representatives of the public or local opinion. They sit for a specified length of time and are given information to help with the decision making process. As in a real jury, experts are asked to give evidence and jurors have the opportunity to ask questions and debate issues.
- *User consultation panels*: they are made up of local people who are selected to represent the local population. Membership is rotated to ensure a broad range of views. Topics for discussion are decided in advance and members have access to the relevant information. These meetings may be facilitated by a moderator (Bowie *et al.*, 1995).

- *Focus groups*: semi-structured discussion with a group of no more than eight participants. These are led by a moderator and are focused on specific topics. Discussion is encouraged.
- *Questionnaire surveys*: these can be postal or distributed by practitioners. This method provides a structured systematic approach to data collection from a large population sample. It does not, however, allow for discussion and assumes a certain level of knowledge from participants.
- *Opinion surveys of standing panels*: these are a sociologically representative sample (usually more than 100) of the population. People are surveyed for their views at intervals and membership is changed after a specific time.
- *Established community nursing contact*: nurses are already in touch with local networks such as community associations, mother and toddler groups and voluntary organizations and should utilize these contacts to enhance the process of user participation in health needs assessment.
- *Public Board meetings*: it is a requirement for board meetings (for both PCGs and trusts) to be held in public and in this way members of the community, although not able to participate at the meeting, can be fully informed of progress and specific decisions made about local health care provision.

Planning for health needs assessment

Health needs assessment, by its very nature, is a complex process, therefore it requires an organized approach to its planning and implementation. Johnstone (1999) describes three steps to assessing health need (Figure 3.3), they are:

- *Step 1*
  Define the population and its boundaries.
  Look at routine data from different sources.
- *Step 2*
  Involve the general public and service users.
  Gain an overview of health and social need.
  Prioritize those areas requiring more detailed and in-depth analysis.
- *Step 3*
  Analyse some areas in more detail. For example, this could be either a disease, a client group or a particular speciality.
  Make recommendations for changes to current provision using a range of data sources, including epidemiology, best practice and research and evidence-based practice.
  Identify how these recommendations could be resourced.

Eleven questions for assessing health needs

It has already been established that the current health agenda or recent research may determine the parameters of the health needs assessment exercise. Therefore, it may be helpful to answer the following questions when

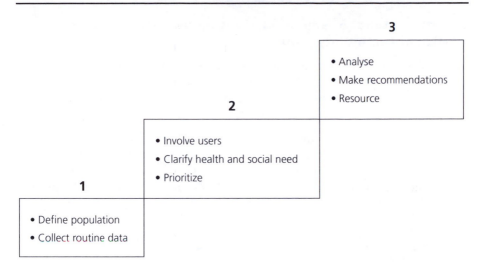

Figure 3.3 The three steps of health needs assessment

embarking on an assessment of need. In order to give a practical application to these questions the following scenario will be used.

The health visiting service is currently being reviewed in line with the recommendations of *Making a Difference* (DOH, 1999b) and *Saving Lives* (DOH, 1999a) and therefore the health needs of the population in the area must be assessed in order to inform the future development of that service.

Question 1 What is the aim of the assessment?

- Does it address a specific agenda whereby the aims are clearly identified?
- What is that agenda?
- Has it a specified resource or time limit?

The agenda is clearly determined by the fact that there must be a more team-centred, public health approach to health visiting in the future. The expectation is that this should be achieved within the next five years and there is no additional funding to support this development.

Question 2 Who is the community to be assessed?

- Have they got specific characteristics?
- Do they access specific health care services?
- Why have they been identified?

This may need to have some further clarification but there is clearly an expectation that the community under consideration should not be confined to the pre-school population, which may have been the case in the past. Are there specific groups within the community which should be targeted and why?

Question 3 What or who are the resources available to this particular community/group?

- Who are the professionals who have contact with this community/group?
- What range of services is accessible to this community/group?
- Are there specific issues relating to meeting the needs of this community?
- What services are already available and well-evaluated?

This will involve a consideration of the current provision of the health visitor service, together with an evaluation or audit of that provision, applying recent literature and research to the analysis. Health and social data relating to the client group will need to be collated in order to determine the priority areas of need.

Question 4 What forum would bring together the key stakeholders?

- Are there already established groups which could be utilized for this exercise?
- Does a new group have to be established?
- Who is best to take the lead and why?

How do the health visitors currently involve their clients or the community in decisions about the provision of care? This exercise may raise specific questions about the appropriateness of the current health visiting service. This may result in specific groups and other agencies being consulted about their perceptions of health need.

Question 5 What is the agreed plan of action?

- Which/who is the most appropriate agency/person to do this?
- Does this require a joint approach?
- Will there be a leader/co-ordinator?
- Is there a timescale?

Is there a project leader or named health visitor to lead on this initiative? The use of an experienced community nurse, who can be seconded to this type of activity may be invaluable. First, it ensures practitioners are actively involved in any proposed changes to their service and, second, it provides an ideal opportunity for individual professional development.

Question 6 What routine data is available?

- What information do we already have?
- What specific information do we need?
- Where can we get it from?

Access to the data routinely collected by health visitors will give some idea of the health-visiting activity, in addition to the more centrally collected population data. However, this exercise should also uncover the gaps in the service and the data collection which need to be addressed in any future development. For example, is there information about out-of-hours GP visits to children under five, which may indicate the need for a more flexible and responsive health-visiting service within the area?

Question 7 How can we involve other agencies and the users?

- Are there any legal or ethical issues involved in collecting data?
- Is joint working already established?

Health visitors, in common with other community nurses, have a wide network of contacts and it is important to recognize existing structures rather than reinventing the wheel. This exercise can be used to identify those agencies where there are little or no formal links with the health visitors.

Question 8 How can we prioritize?

- What are the criteria?
- How do we decide on the criteria?

This will need a clear reference to the overall recommendations for the health visiting service as identified in *Making a Difference* (DOH, 1999b) in conjunction with the local HImP and workforce planning initiative.

Question 9 Are there additional areas for consideration?

- Why is this an area of recognized need?
- Can we utilize work already completed as evidence?
- What additional surveys do we need to undertake?

This may identify the need for additional exploratory work in line with local and national activity.

Question 10 Once the data has been collected and analysed, who can act upon the recommendations?

- Do we need to do any additional networking?
- Do we need to access expert help advice or support?

The key stakeholders should be consulted and informed of the proposed developments to the health visiting service. The need for close collaboration is essential within the development of PCTs.

Question 11 What is the plan for action?

- What happens next?
- By whom?

- In what time?
- What are the expected outcomes?
- How do we know we have reached them?
- How many resources will we need?
- How much funding is available?
- What are the short and long term implications for the defined population?

It is essential that a clear plan of action is identified on completion of the assessment process.

This exercise has demonstrated how a logical and systematic approach to health needs assessment can be achieved, particularly if there is a specific purpose or goal. In order to illustrate this still further, the next section will relate to a real-life health needs assessment project. It illustrates how inter-agency collaboration enhances and informs a needs assessment within a defined population, while addressing an explicit policy agenda, which in this case was for Sure Start. The names of the locations within this case study have been changed but the data collected represents the actual information contained within the three-month project report.

Case study

ASSESSING HEALTH NEEDS IN MIDDLETOWN

In December 1998, representatives from a range of statutory and voluntary agencies in Middletown met to discuss the possibility of a Sure Start programme (Home Office, 1999) within the area. The membership included representation from:

- The community NHS Trust.
- The acute hospital NHS Trust (community children's nursing service).
- The children's information centre.
- A consultant paediatrician.
- The educational psychological service.
- The early years learning centre.
- The Health Authority.
- The PCG.
- Homestart.
- The midwifery service
- Parents and Children Together (PACT).
- Policy and planning department.
- Social services, children and families.
- Youth and community service.

It was felt that these people represented the services which had the greatest impact upon the outcomes identified in the Sure Start initiative. It was agreed at the initial meeting that there was potential within Middletown to develop a Sure Start programme, but in order to address the criteria and establish the needs of a specific community, more detailed information was required. A health visitor was seconded to carry out an initial needs assessment of Middletown to inform the selection of a potential site and it was envisaged that this work would also inform the future application process. The health visitor seconded to the project was also the specialist health visitor for the homeless in the area and her role had retained a well-defined public health perspective of health care. The skills and working practices developed within this specialist role were invaluable to this project as she had already established effective collaborative links with the voluntary and statutory agencies within the town. This provided access to a wide range of information sources.

Note: In this instance, although there was always a recognized and well-documented health and social need in Middletown, it was the Sure Start initiative which focused this specific health needs assessment process. It was the political and/or policy agenda which determined both the *need* and the *demand* (see Figure 3.1) in this case and the area for action was therefore determined by identifying the need in relation to the prescribed policy agenda.

To recapitulate, Sure Start is part of the government's strategy to reduce inequalities by improving services to families within a designated area by the provision of a more co-ordinated approach to health and social care. There are clearly defined targets to be achieved within a Sure Start programme and these, in turn, inform both the needs and the demands of the assessment process. Table 3.1 demonstrates the extent to which need and demand is determined by the policy agenda.

MIDDLETOWN

Middletown is a thriving commercial centre in the Home Counties. The common perception of the area is that the town's residents have a lifestyle of affluence. The reality is that increased demand for housing has forced up prices and private sector rents are now way beyond the means of those on average incomes. This has led to increased homelessness in the area and the occupation of substandard, private sector accommodation by those on a low income. It has also concentrated the occupation of social housing clusters by the least-able. It was felt that these pockets of deprivation would benefit from Sure Start resources.

The 11 questions detailed above were used to provide a framework and a systematic approach for the health needs assessment of Middletown.

ASSESSING THE HEALTH NEEDS OF MIDDLETOWN

Question 1 What is the aim of the assessment?

To identify an area whose health and social needs matched the Sure Start criteria (see Table 3.1). The assessment had to be completed within three months to meet the Sure Start timescale.

Table 3.1 The needs and demands of a Sure Start programme

Needs	Demands
To improve information and support to parents*	An outreach and home visiting service*
To reduce the number of children on the child protection register	More health and social support for families*
To support mothers with post-natal depression*	Improved health and social care provision*
To reduce low birthweight babies by 5%*	Improved support for children with special needs*
To ensure normal speech and language development in 90% of children*	Affordable child care
To ensure access to good quality play and learning*	Support for holidays and outings
To encourage parental representation*	More locally based services
To improve the quality of services*	A community cafe
	Better transport provision

*Stated objectives of the Sure Start programme

Question 2 Which is the community to be assessed?

There was a need to identify the area of Middletown that most closely resembled the criteria laid down by Sure Start. This involved a systematic analysis of available data with the emphasis on young families and deprivation, hence the inclusion of information for *housing and amenities, social class, employment, ethnicity and children per household*. Much of the information related to political wards within the town.

Through networking it was discovered that Census data for each political ward was available from the Middletown planning department. The figures (Table 3.2) refer to Middletown as a whole (italic print denotes the political ward(s) with the highest rates).

DEPRIVATION INDICES

The Jarman Index uses dependency indicators, devised initially to demonstrate the workload of family doctors. The total score denotes the level of deprivation in an area and the intensity of the GPs' workload.

The planning department also provided a plan of the town depicting the Jarman scores of the political wards. Of the 15 political wards, the six with the highest Jarman score and therefore the highest levels of deprivation were:

- Kimble 43.
- Merton 37.

- Amber 27.
- Bart 26.
- Chalfont 20.
- Winston 19.

Perusal of the government's *Guide for Trailblazers Sure Start* (Home Office, 1999) indicated that the *Index of Local Deprivation* (DETR, 1998) was the preferred evidence of need for Sure Start. This was not readily available to the project health visitor and a search on the internet revealed that the index incorporated a range of deprivation indices. All the electoral wards in England have been ranked in order of deprivation. The most-deprived being ranked one and the least-deprived 8689. The ranking of the three most-deprived wards of Middletown was:

- Amber 258.
- Kimble 610.
- Winston 771.

It was discovered that this information is available at enumeration district level. An enumeration district is the geographical area covered by one Census data recording officer. Enumeration districts are smaller than political wards, there being 8689 political wards in England compared with 66 716 enumeration districts. It can be very time-consuming and costly to access this information. Discussions with local authority staff revealed that this information was readily available from the local planning department. Further questioning with staff in various departments of the Borough Council enabled the index scores for enumeration districts to be mapped across the town. There were 21 enumeration districts in the town having a rank lower than 10 000. The lowest ranking areas were in Winston and Netly.

ANALYSIS AND PRIORITIZATION OF NEED

A review of the data thus far indicated that the areas of highest need according to:

- Census data were Winston, Amber and Bart.
- The Jarman index were Kimble, Amber, Bart and Winston.
- The index of local deprivation were Amber, Kimble and Winston.
- The poorest ward was Winston (adjacent to Kimble).
- The most-featured wards were Amber and Bart.

Therefore, the two possible areas for Sure Start were identified as:

- Winston: an area incorporating parts of Winston and Kimble which had the greatest concentration of social housing in the town.
- Netly: an area covering parts of Amber and Bart with much of the housing stock old and privately rented and with great cultural diversity among its residents.

As two the areas of Winston and Netly had been identified for further scrutiny, the next step was to undertake a comparative needs assessment.

Table 3.2 Selected Census data (ONS, 1991)

Housing tenure	(% of households)	Highest-rated wards
Owner-occupied	67%	*Thyme*
Private	14%	*Amber*
Rented	19%	*Winston*
Amenities		
No car	33%	*Amber/Winston*
Overcrowded	2%	*Winston*
Lacking/sharing bathroom WC	2.5%	*Amber/Bart*
No central heating	19%	*Kimble Amber and Bart*
Social class		
Professional	11%	*Thyme*
Managerial	31%	*Thyme*
Skilled non-manual	15%	*Catley*
Skilled manual	25%	*Turton*
Partially skilled	11%	*North*
Manual	6%	*Winston*
Ethnicity		
White	91%	*Thyme/Turton*
Black	4%	*Bart*
Asian	4%	*Bart/Amber*
Children		
Children aged under 4	7%	*Bart/Winston*
Lone-parent families	4%	*Winston*
Dependent children	28%	*Winston*
3+ Dependent children	6%	*Winston*
4+ Dependent children	2%	*Winston*
Unemployment		
Percentage of males aged 16–59 years	9%	*Winston*
Percentage of females 16–59 years	4%	*Amber and Winston*

Question 3 What or who are the resources available to the community?

The aims of Sure Start are to add value to existing services and to promote a partnership approach. It seemed logical therefore, to identify and map local resources (Table 3.3) and to contact potential partners. Written information and interviews were requested from:

- Heads of primary schools.
- Youth and community staff.
- Family centre staff.
- Community nurses and health visitors.
- Parents attending child health clinics.

Table 3.3 clearly demonstrates the wide range of information available within a community which can inform health needs assessment. It is also clear that a focus on a specific area of need enables practitioners to work collaboratively and thus accumulate a wealth of information to address a specific agenda. It also enables community nurses to work in partnership with other agencies to assist with resource mapping and to clarify future collaborative working.

Question 4 What forum would bring together the stakeholders?

The forum for this particular health needs assessment had already been established but the process can form an impetus for future collaboration and partnership working within the community. There were already two successful partnerships within these communities. A single regeneration budget building scheme in Netly had already acquired funding and there was a project currently being drafted in Winston. In true partnership spirit, it was agreed that the link to a potential Sure Start scheme would be included in the Winston bid. Reciprocally, a bid for Sure Start funding would state the connection to the regeneration budget.

The partnership approach flourished when this connection led to meeting the education action zone planning team. The project nurse became a temporary team member and wrote a section of the bid relating to Sure Start. The two single regeneration budget projects and the education action zone plans would provide equitably for Winston and Netly.

Information was gathered with the assistance of the initiative group which collaborated in sharing information and locating other sources. The spirit of co-operation and collaboration continued among all those who were approached for information. This was a reciprocal process, not only in the inclusion in the bidding process for different projects but in the two-way exchange and the level of co-operation and degree of enthusiasm expressed by everyone that was approached.

Question 5 What is the agreed plan of action?

Once agreement had been reached on the chosen area for the Sure Start programme, the initiative group was to contact the Sure Start unit to inform them

Table 3.3 Identifying and contacting local resources

Resource	Source	Method
Preschool education	Social Services	By telephone
Toddler groups	Section 19	Referred to agent
Playgroups	Annual review	Children's information centre
Nurseries	Day care	Telephone and document
Primary schools	Local knowledge	School nurses
Primary school league tables	Library	Department of Education publication
School breakfast clubs	Head teachers	Interview
After-school clubs	Town children's	Request from source
Language in schools	Local authority	Telephone request
Adult literacy classes	Head teachers	Interview
Free school meals	Local authority	Telephone request
Family centres	Social services	Telephone
Community centres	Local knowledge	Telephone
Health centres	Local knowledge	Contact local community NHS Trust
GP surgeries	Health authority	Telephone
(alternatively)	Community health council	Telephone
Views of potential partners	Networking	Interviews
Level of local interest	Community nurses	Group consultation
Clinic users	Straw poll	
Social services	Social services	Written information
Community health statistics	NHS line manager	Personal request
Single regeneration projects	Borough council	Meeting with staff
Education action	Borough council	Meeting with staff
Health action zone project	Borough council	Meeting with staff
Crime statistics	Community safety audit document	Networking Telephone

of the health needs assessment process which had enabled that decision to be made.

Questions 6 and 7 What routine data is available? How can we involve other agencies and users?

Census and local data had already been collected to inform the decision-making process. However, there was still further data which needed to be collected, specific to the criteria of Sure Start. This included information about education, ethnicity, language, special needs, free school meals, child protection and crime. The project health visitor worked closely with other agencies to obtain this information (Table 3.4).

Education

With the exception of Church School, all attained below average in the Level 4 tests in 1998 and 1999 (Department of Education, 1998/99). The Winston scores are lower than Netly, and half the Winston pupils are in educational need, compared to Netly with less than one-third (DE, 1998) which suggest greater educational need in Winston.

Ethnicity

The percentage of ethnic minority populations in Winston and Netly, each of which covers parts of two electoral wards, was calculated from the Census data (ONS, 1991) (Table 3.5).

Table 3.4 Education data specific to Sure Start critieria

| School | Average no. of pupils | | Special educational needs | |
	1998	1999	With Statement	No Statement
Winston Grange	36	194	7	98
Winston Park	29	401	11	215
Netly	52	369	8	95
Church	65	252	6	57

Table 3.5 Ethnic origins (%) of populations in Winston and Netley

Ethnic origins	Winston	Netly
White	90%	80%
Pakistani	2.5%	7.5%
Indian	1%	2.8%
Afro-Caribbean	3%	5.5%

Language

It was shown that pupils in Winston achieved less than those in Netley, despite the greater majority of children having English as a first language (Table 3.6).

Free school meals

Information on free school meals was obtained from the local authority education department (Table 3.7).

The lower percentage of free school meal claims in Netly might be interpreted as lesser economic need. However, Census details (ONS, 1991) may be used to calculate the average unemployment rates for Winston and Netly; these are 12% and 10%, respectively. The reason for the lower percentage of claimants in Netly might be linguistic and cultural, rather than economic, including lack of information in an understandable format, a greater sense of pride or concerns about the cultural acceptance of foods prepared away from home. Attention to cross-cultural information might encourage uptake of services due, such as free school meals, thereby contributing to relieving poverty.

Crime

Crime statistics are relevant to the Sure Start aims of supporting parents, promoting educational achievement and preventing social exclusion.

As a requirement of the Crime and Disorder Act (Home Office,1998b) Middletown Borough Council, in partnership with the local police department, produced a community safety audit. The average crime rate for Winston was in excess of ten per 100 head of population and that of Netly less than six per 100 head of population. The number of youth offenders per 100 population of young people is 2.8 in Winston and less than one per 100 population of young people in Netly.

Table 3.6 Percentage of school children whose first language is not English

Winston		Netly	
Winston Park	4%	Church	No data
Winston Grange	17%	Netly	56%

Table 3.7 Percentage of children claiming free school meals

Winston		Netly	
Winston Park	37.5%	Church	No data
	(79 children)	(—)	
Winston Grange	46%	Netly	25.5%
	(74 children)	(63 children)	

Child protection

The community safety audit also recorded the numbers of children on the child protection register and those 'looked after' by social services.

For child protection, the rate per 100 head of population in the police sector covering Winston is double that of the sector around Netly, at 0.04 and 0.02 per 100 head of population, respectively. 'Looked after' children refers to those whose accommodation is supervised by social services and can include children's homes, supported accommodation, trustee care or support at home. The Winston area has a rate for 'looked after' children in excess of 0.15 per 100 head of population, whereas the rate for Netly has a lower rate of less than 0.05 per 100 head of population.

Question 8 How can we prioritize?

The data showed that in many respects there was little difference in the needs of the two areas identified. Economically, the two areas were similar and the statutory community resources were comparable within each area. Educational achievement seemed equally poor for the pupils resident in each area (Department of Education, 1998/1999).

However, in addition to poor educational performance, Winston had a larger percentage of children with special educational needs, which might indicate that the need for additional support is greater. The general crime rate and the rate of youth offenders were also higher in Winston; this suggested that the likelihood of social exclusion was more likely. These are specifically the types of problem that Sure Start (Home Office, 1999) seeks to address.

The numbers of children on the child protection register and the numbers of those 'looked after' by social services was much higher in Winston. Again, this indicated that the level of deprivation is higher in Winston.

The comments of teachers, at interview, reiterated the choice of Winston as the chosen area for the Sure Start project. The teachers in Netly were concerned about linguistic and cultural issues, whereas the teachers in Winston were concerned about pupils' poor state of nutrition, small stature, poor health, incidence of disabilities and psychological problems. These are issues that depict an area of great deprivation and one that the Sure Start initiative seeks to address. Thus, Winston was duly selected by the multi-agency initiative group.

Question 9 Are there additional areas for consideration?

Although sufficient data was presented for Winston to be selected as a potential site for a project, the time in which the work had to be completed was very short and therefore the range of the consultation process was limited. Therefore, further work must be done to identify partners in service provision to manage the project and decide the form in which it will exist, how its services will be located and delivered. Most importantly, further needs assessment should include the views of the residents. It was felt by the initiative group that it would be ethically unacceptable to interview residents and raise expectations for a project that may not be placed in that community. It was agreed that once any funding had been identified they would be consulted for their views and opinions.

These sources might include focus groups with local residents and potential service users, toddler groups, playgroups or nurseries. It is hoped that other groups of practitioners and managers of statutory and voluntary agencies might be consulted in focus groups. Additional statutory practitioners might include representatives of all relevant community nurse groups, PCG representatives, paramedics, social services and a greater range of voluntary service providers.

Question 10 Who can act on the recommendations?

The group was informed in November 1999 that Middletown had been named as one of the sites for the second wave for Sure Start. Outline plans were to be submitted by February 2000, with final implementation plans to be submitted in May 2000. This initiated a full consultation process with the community of Winston which had not been addressed in the original work.

Question 11 What is the plan of action?

The programme has now moved to its final and most challenging stage: that of planning and implementation. This process in itself is worthy of another chapter. The current challenges now facing the Sure Start project team in Middletown include:

- The realities of partnership working with the statutory and voluntary agencies and the community itself.
- Encouraging the community to engage in and own the project.
- Difficult decisions about capital development projects.
- Issues concerning general organizational and project management.

Conclusion

Health needs assessment is a key characteristic of the current health care agenda. However, the current emphasis upon partnership working, user involvement and a reduction of inequality has given rise to a more policy-driven approach to the assessment of health and social need. Practitioners and agencies must work together more effectively to pool resources and expertise, to assemble information and inform future health and social care within the community. The Middletown case study has provided an excellent example of how different agencies can work together to achieve this. Through working in partnership a wide range of information from a variety of sources was collected, collated and analysed. It was then used to identify the needs of the population within a defined geographical area. The resultant report was then used to attract funding for future activity. It also served the dual purpose of identifying ways in which agencies could better work together in the future.

The Introduction to this chapter stated that health needs assessment was a difficult concept to define. The definition may be difficult and the process itself can be challenging but effective health needs assessment can result in an improvement in working relationships and more importantly it can make a real difference to the health and life chances of those living in the community.

References

Bowie, C., Richardson, A. and Sykes, W. (1995) Consulting the public about health care priorities. *British Medical Journal*, 311: 1168–9.

Bradshaw, J. (1972) The concept of social need. *New Society*, 30: 640–3.

Department of Health (DOH). (1987) *Promoting better health*. London: HMSO.

Department of Health (DOH). (1989) *Working for patients*. London: HMSO.

Department of Health (DOH). (1990) *The National Health Service and community care act*. London: HMSO.

Department of Health (DOH). (1992) *The health of the nation*. London: HMSO.

Department of Health (DOH). (1997) *The New NHS – modern and dependable*. London: HMSO.

Department of Health (DOH). (1998) *Report of the independent inquiry into inequalities in health*. London: HMSO.

Department of Health (DOH). (1999a) *Saving lives: our healthier nation*. London: The Stationery Office.

Department of Health (DOH). (1999b) *Making a difference*. London: The Stationery Office.

Fatchett, A. (1998) *Nursing in the new NHS: modern and dependable?* London: Bailliere Tindall.

Hall, D. (1996) *Health for all children*. Oxford: Oxford University Press.

Hipkin, L, Dixon, M. and Smith, P. (1999) The contribution of nurses, commissioning and fundholding GPs. In: *The PCG development guide*. Oxford: Radcliffe Medical Press.

Home Office. (1998a) *Supporting families*. London: HMSO.

Home Office. (1998b) *Crime and disorder act*. London: HMSO.

Home Office. (1999) *A guide for trailblazers Sure Start*. London: HMSO.

Jarman, B. (1983) Identification of underprivileged areas. *British Medical Journal*, 286: 1006.

Johnstone, P. (1999) Health needs assessment and health improvement programmes. In: *The PCG development guide*. Oxford: Radcliffe Medical Press.

Jordan, J., Wright, J., Wilkinson, J. and Williams, R. (1998) Assessing local health needs in primary care: understanding and experience in three English districts. *Quality in Health Care*, 7: 83–9.

Kilduff, A., McKeown, K. and Crowther, A. (1998) Health needs assessment in primary care: the evolution of a practical public health approach. *Public Health*, 112: 175–81.

Kings Fund Pace Project. (1998) *Improving the care of patients with leg ulcers*. London: Kings Fund.

Moffatt, C. and Dolman, M. (1995) recurrence of leg ulcers within a community ulcer service. *Journal of Wound Care*, 4: 56–62.

Percy Smith, J. and Sanderson, I. (1992) *Understanding local needs*. London: Institute for Public Policy Research.

Stevens, A. and Gabbay, J. (1991) Needs assessment needs assessment. *Health Trends*, 23: 20–3.

Stevens, A. and Gillam, S. (1998) Needs assessment: from theory to practice. *British Medical Journal*, 316: 1448–52.

Stevens, A. and Raftery, J. (1997) Introduction. In: *Health care needs assessment, the epidemiologically based needs assessment reviews*. Oxford: Radcliffe Medical Press.

Tinson, S. (1995) Assessing health need: a community perspective. In: Cain, P., Hyde, V. and Howkins, E. (eds) *Community nursing: dimensions and dilemmas*. London: Arnold.

Whitehead, M. (1992) The health divide. In: Townsend, P. and Davidson, N. (eds) *Inequalities in health*. Harmondsworth: Penguin.

Williams, R. and Wright, J. (1998) Epidemiological issues in health needs assessment *British Medical Journal*, 316: 1819–23.

SOURCES OF INFORMATION FOR HEALTH NEEDS ASSESSMENT:

Department of Education. (1998) *Primary school league tables*. London: The Stationery Office.

Department of Education. (1999) *Primary school league tables*. London: HMSO.

Department of Social Security (DHSS). (1996) *Population estimates*. London: Office National Statistics.

Department of the Environment, Transport and Regions (DETR). (1993) *Total land area*. London: DETR.

Department of the Environment, Transport and Regions (DETR). (1998) *Index of local deprivation*. London: The London Research Centre.

Department for Education and Employment (DfEE). (1996) *Population estimates*. London: Office National Statistics.

Department of Education (DE). (1998) *Primary school league tables*. London: HMSO.

Department of Education (DE). (1999) *Primary school league tables*. London: HMSO.

Norwich Union, Royal and Sun Alliance and United Assurance. (1997) *Home insurance weightings*. London: Norwich Union, Royal and Sun Alliance and United Assurance.

Nationwide Building Society. (1989) *Local housing statistics 1*. England: Nationwide Building Society.

NOMIS. (1997) *Population estimates*. London: Office National Statistics.

ONS. (1991) *Census*. London: The Stationery Office.

Providing community care to individuals with mental health problems

4

Mary Watkins

Introduction

It is now common for individuals to receive mental health care, support and treatment in a community environment (Brooker and Repper, 1998). This change has been achieved over the last 30 years. Until the 1970s, most treatment for individuals suffering severe and recurring mental health illness was provided within inpatient facilities. The challenges to community health and social care workers have increased as inpatient facilities have gradually reduced and individuals with mental health problems have been able to lead much more normal lives in community settings with appropriate treatment and support provided in a range of facilities (Falloon and Faddon, 1993; Strathdee and Sutherby, 1996; Brooker and Repper, 1998).

Range and specification of care provision for users

Facilities vary widely across the four countries within the UK and, indeed, between health authorities. In Northern Ireland, mental health services are provided under a health and social care structure that promotes comprehensive health and social care service for individuals. This approach is currently being piloted in England in Somerset, where a new partnership Trust was set up in 1998. The Somerset Partnership NHS Trust is attempting to provide seamless services for individuals with mental health problems. More commonly, however, inpatient facilities are provided by the health service, either in acute trusts or in community-orientated NHS Trusts, with aftercare for individuals who have received inpatient treatment being provided through community care facilities. A proportion of individuals, for example psychiatrists and mental health nurses, are being employed by Trusts, with social workers being employed in social services. At times, it has been recognized that effective co-ordination of mental health services has been very difficult to achieve with different employers for health and social care professionals. In some instances, users come into contact with three or four agencies that, as a result of managerial organization, do not necessarily have adequate structures for communication to ensure structured supervision in the community (DOH, 1996; Lucas, 1996; Peck, 1998). It is now recognized that it is imperative to achieve integration and consistency of care for people with mental health problems in the community.

THE NATIONAL HEALTH SERVICE FRAMEWORK FOR MENTAL HEALTH

Since the introduction of the care planning approach (CPA) (DOH, 1994; SSI and NHS Executive, 1999), the *Mental Health National Service Framework* has been produced by the Department of Health for England (DOH, 1999).

The Introduction to this document by the then Secretary of State for Health, Frank Dobson, reminds us that at any one time one adult in six is suffering from some form of mental illness. In other words, mental illness is as common as asthma. The Foreword clarifies that there is a wide range of mental illness within the population, including common conditions such as anxiety and depression, and more complex illnesses, such as schizophrenia, which affect fewer than one person in 100. This document states that despite the prevalence and importance of mental illness, structures to ensure adequate care provision for all those with mental health problems have not had the attention that has been deserved, a concept held by several texts on the subject, including Brooker and Repper (1998). The government has therefore decided to identify national standards for mental health, which should be developed, achieved and delivered within the next decade. The standards have been founded on a sound basis of research evidence as a result of work conducted by an external reference group. The fact that the standards are evidence-based should not be minimized as it has been argued that too much health care delivery has been based on 'belief' rather than on research-based evidence (DOH, 1991). If the National Health Service (NHS) framework for mental health is to be adequately achieved, the next ten years should see the gradual development and improvement of mental health services in the community, based on current and newly developed evidence. The guiding values and principles of the *Mental Health National Service Framework* (DOH, 1999) may appear simplistic but are, in fact, quite revolutionary in terms of placing users and the carers of those using services as the central focus of developments. The framework, written in the form of a user's compact, states that:

. . . people with mental health problems can expect that services will:

- involve services users and their carers in planning and delivery of care
- deliver high quality and treatment of care which is known to be effective and acceptable
- be well-suited to those who use them and non-discriminatory
- be accessible so that help can be obtained when and where it is needed
- promote their safety and that of their carers and wider public
- offer choices which promote independence

- be well co-ordinated between all staff and agencies
- deliver continuity of care for as long as it is needed
- empower and support their staff
- be properly accountable to the public, service, users and carers.

(DOH, 1999: 4)

These principles and values should guide all individuals working with users of mental health services, whether those users are suffering from a short depressive illness that responds rapidly to treatment, or have been diagnosed as having a recurring illness which includes psychotic elements, sometimes necessitating compulsory treatment under the Mental Health Act. To date user empowerment has been acknowledged as desirable (MIND, 1983, 1993a, 1993b; Campbell, 1989; DOH, 1994), but has never been so clearly defined as a necessity within service development as within the national service framework.

USERS' INVOLVEMENT IN SELECTING TREATMENT

There will, of course, be times when it is very difficult to achieve the standards outlined in the *Mental Health National Service Framework* (DOH, 1999), particularly in terms of patients having real choice in relation to treatment and accessibility (Lucas, 1996; Morgan, 1998). To date, innovative mental health services tend to have developed from a bottom-up approach in response to either innovations from professionals or demands from local focus and user groups. It is quite clear, when talking to users of a variety of services across the country, that some feel that they do not have access to psychotherapy in community care; others believe that they are not being prescribed the most effective psychotropic drugs, this being based on cost rather than on effectiveness decisions. It is interesting to note that the NHS framework anticipates that care provision should in future be based predominantly on evidence. Sometimes, however, evidence collected through randomized control trials illustrates that services may not necessarily be cost effective (NHS Centre for Reviews and Dissemination, 1997, 1999). However, this does not mean that individuals with particular mental health problems do not value those services. It is, for example, well recognized that individuals with cancer may seek to have aromatherapy and massage funded through a state system. There is little doubt that both these interventions provide a relief to individuals, but whether they are cost effective in comparison to certain cancer drugs remains a difficult question to answer. The pressure from individuals in cancer services has, however, often resulted in these services being available on the NHS. There is an increasingly strong mental health lobby demanding, for example, that psychotherapy should be available to individuals with psychotic illness during periods when they are relatively well. There is little doubt that psychotherapy assists individuals to understand their illness and may, in some respects, result in them 'feeling better' for a period. Whether psychotherapy is cost effective in relation to health care outcomes in comparison to certain psychotropic drugs and psycho-educational programmes remains a major question (Kagan *et al.*, 1992; Caplin *et al.*, 1997; Kemp *et al.*, 1998; NHS Centre for Reviews and Dissemination, 1999).

The commitment to considering users' and carers' views on *'supportive'* service provision reflects previous direction, recognizing that it is necessary to provide supportive services for patients and service users, their families and carers, to build healthier communities. An adequate definition of 'supportive services' is one that may be increasingly necessary over the next decade as individual health care practitioners try to provide services for users and carers. It is possible that users' and carers' perceptions of what should be provided to support them, may exceed the resources allocated.

PRIMARY CARE STANDARDS FOR THE NHS FRAMEWORK FOR MENTAL HEALTH

Standards two and three within the framework (DOH, 1999) are particularly orientated towards primary care and access to services for individuals. The aim of these standards is 'to deliver better primary mental health care and to ensure consistent advice and help for people with mental health needs, including primary care services for individuals with severe mental illness'. Standards two and three are detailed in Table 4.1.

The challenge to health care professionals, in terms of working with individuals in the community, is to turn these standards into reality and to provide consistent advice and seamless services to users in rural and urban settings. The findings of a variety of inquiries, including those regarding Christopher Clunis (Ritchie *et al.*, 1994) and Ms Justine Cummings (Somerset Health Authority and Social Services, 2000), illustrate that often individual users fall through a

Table 4.1   Primary care standards from the NHS framework for mental health (DOH, 1999)

Aim
To deliver better primary mental health care and to ensure consistent advice and help for people with mental health needs, including primary care services for individuals with severe mental illness

Standard two
Any service users who contact their primary health care team with a common mental health problem should:

> have their mental health needs identified and assessed

> be offered effective treatments, including referral to specialist services for further assessment, treatment and care if they require it

Standard three
Any individual with a common mental health problem should:

> be able to make contact round the clock with local services necessary to meet their needs and receive adequate care

> be able to use NHS Direct, as it develops, for first-level advice and referral on to specialist helplines and local services

monitoring net, not through any lack of commitment from health and social care staff to the concept of support and advice, but rather through a lack of co-ordination of care (Morgan, 1998). It is anticipated that access to specialist services will be provided in the future through ready accessibility in that:

> A duty doctor, Section 12 approved, and an approved social worker must be available around the clock, every day of the year. Services should provide a more comprehensive approach, with better access to the multi-disciplinary mental health team for emergency assessment and care. All local agencies, including the police, need to be able to access specialist mental health services, including secure psychiatric services, for 24 hours a day.
>
> (DOH, 1999: 33).

In order to achieve standards two and three, each primary care group (PCG) or primary care trust (PCT) will be expected to work with specialist mental health services to develop resources within each practice to assess mental health needs and to work with diverse groups in the population. Teams will be required to develop skills and competencies to manage common mental health problems and to agree *transparent* arrangements for referring individuals for assessment, advice or treatment. Perhaps the greatest challenge is that each PCG will be expected to have the skills and necessary organizational systems to provide the full range of health care identified in care plans for people with severe mental illness. This should include physical health care and other primary care support as identified necessary for individuals.

To achieve standards two and three each PCG or PCT will need to work with the support of specialist mental health services to:

- Develop the resources within each practice to assess mental health needs.
- Develop the resources to work with diverse groups in the population.
- Develop the skills and competencies to manage common mental health problems.
- Agree the arrangements for referral for assessment, advice or treatment and care.
- Have the skills and the necessary organizational systems to provide the physical health care and other primary care support needed, as agreed in their care plan, for people with severe mental illness.

The care programme approach

It is widely recognized that health and social care workers need to work towards providing an integrated approach to the support, supervision and treatment of users of mental health services. It is suggested that the seamless provision of services could be more consistently achieved with an integrated approach to care co-ordination across health and social care providers.

A Social Services Inspectorate (SSI) and NHS Executive policy booklet (SSI and NHS Executive, 1999), *Effective Care Co-ordination in Mental Health Services*, refers to modernizing the care programme approach (CPA). An understanding of this document is important for people who are involved with providing care for individuals with mental health problems in community settings. Broadly, the context is as follows:

- The government requires the NHS and social services to work in partnership to provide integrated services that will improve the quality of life for all citizens.
- Services should be accessible and should intervene more quickly to offer healthcare and social support, seeking out those who are difficult to engage, involve users and carers in planning developments, and use effective care processes to be delivered in partnership across health and social care as well as other agencies.
- Recognition is given to the fact that individuals' mental health problems place demands on services that no one discipline or agency can meet alone. It is therefore now government policy that a system of effective co-ordination is required for all services to benefit the service user. A range of services is referred to within the document, including housing, finance, employment, education and physical health needs, in addition to mental health and social care.

There are four main elements to the CPA which was first introduced in 1991:

- Systematic arrangements for assessing the health and social needs of people accepted into special mental health services.
- The formation of a care plan which identifies the health and social care required from a variety of providers.
- The appointment of a key worker to keep in close touch with the service user and to monitor and co-ordinate care.
- Regular review and where necessary, agree changes to the care plan (SSI and NHS Executive, 1999: 1).

The CPA to the delivery of health care within a community setting is well established in many areas, based on *Building Bridges* (DOH, 1995). There are formal mechanisms for assessing whether individuals need to be assessed by use of the CPA. The redefinition of the levels of support and monitoring expected for individuals who require long term community care are redefined under Standard four in the *Mental Health National Service Framework* (DOH, 1999). The aim of Standard four is to ensure that all people with severe mental health problems receive a range of services which optimizes their engagement in care provision, anticipates or prevents a crisis and reduces risk to both the individual and their significant others. All mental health users on CPA should have:

- A single point of referral.
- A unified health and social care assessment process.

- Co-ordination of the respective roles and responsibilities of each agency in the system.
- Access, through a single process, to the support and resources of both health and social care (SSI and NHS Executive, 1999).

In order to reduce variation in terms of the definition and application of CPA, it has been redefined in England at two levels 'standard' and 'enhanced' (SSI and NHS Executive, 1999).

STANDARD CPA

Users who are to be classified as requiring standard CPA will normally require the support or intervention of one agency or discipline, and be assessed as posing no danger to themselves or to others, and not to be at high risk if they lose contact with services.

ENHANCED CPA

Individuals who are assessed as requiring enhanced CPA will have more complex care needs and be less likely to engage with services than those requiring standard CPA. Such individuals would need more intensive help from a range of services, and may have more than one clinical condition, or a dual diagnosis of a mental health problem combined with alcohol or drug misuse. Individuals who are assessed as hard to engage, and with whom it is difficult to maintain contact are more likely to require enhanced CPA, particularly if they are assessed as posing a risk if they lost contact with services. Table 4.2 indicates the criteria which should be considered in reaching a decision in relation to providing a user with standard or enhanced CPA.

ASSESSMENT RELATING TO CPA

Once users are defined as requiring CPA it is necessary for a comprehensive assessment of their needs to be undertaken. When conducting such an assessment the following criteria must be considered:

- The nature of any mental health problem experienced by the user.
- Medication that may be prescribed and its potential side effects, and the history of compliance with taking medication.
- The nature of any risk posed and the arrangements for the management of this risk to the service user and to others – carers and the wider public, including the circumstances in which defined contingency action should be taken.
- Any requirement for physical health care: how and what will be provided – usually by the GP, but also by social services when help with meals and personal hygiene may be offered.
- The accessibility and appropriateness of accommodation/housing, appropriate to the service user's needs.

Table 4.2   Characteristics of the CPA (SSI and NHS Executive, 1999)

The characteristics of people on standard CPA will include some of the following:
They require the support or intervention of one agency or discipline or they require only low-key support from more than one agency or discipline
They are more able to self-manage their mental health problems
They have an active informal support network
They pose little danger to themselves or others
They are more likely to maintain appropriate contact with services

People on enhanced CPA are likely to have some of the following characteristics:
They have multiple care needs, including housing, employment, etc., requiring inter-agency co-ordination
They are only willing to co-operate with one professional or agency but they have multiple care needs
They may be in contact with a number of agencies (including the criminal justice system)
They are likely to require more frequent and intensive interventions, perhaps with medication management
They are more likely to have mental health problems co-existing with other problems such as substance misuse
They are more likely to be at risk of harming themselves or others
They are more likely to disengage with services

- Any need for the provision of domestic support actions required to promote employment, education or training or alternative occupation.
- Structures to provide adequate income.
- Provision of cultural and faith needs.
- Structures to promote independence and sustain social contact, including therapeutic leisure activity.

On completion of any comprehensive assessment when a patient is on CPA it is necessary to *agree the date of next planned review*. Although it may be necessary to review an individual's care earlier than the planned date, the provision of a review date should contribute to reducing the possibility of failing to review users' individual care plans on a regular basis.

SUPPORTIVE PARTNERSHIP CENTRAL TO STRUCTURE OF CARE WITHIN CPA

It is expected that care should be structured so that the service provided optimizes users' engagement, anticipates or prevents a crisis and reduces risk of reoccurrence and/or harm to the individual and their significant others. All users on CPA should have a copy of their written care plan, which:

- Includes the action to be taken in a crisis by the service user, the carer and the care co-ordinator.
- Advises GPs how they should respond if the service user needs additional help.
- Has the date of the next anticipated review meeting.

If users are to be well-supported in the community it is essential that mental health services stay in contact with people with severe and enduring mental illness, especially those who are considered to be at risk. In the past, the duty of contact was always seen to be the responsibility of mental health professionals; whereas care co-ordinators are still expected to take on a lead monitoring role and to engage users by providing information in the CPA plan to them, their carers and GPs, responsibility in a crisis may be shared using a partnership approach. For example, a carer may agree to contact the care co-ordinator when a user's health status changes and initiate further intervention. If this is to be achieved, it is essential that clear guidance is given within care plans on how carers and users may access specialist mental health services, 24 hours a day, 365 days a year. Should a crisis develop, users themselves, their carers or GPs should be able to access flexible help and outreach support from mental health services appropriate to their needs.

A named care co-ordinator should be agreed for each user who is to be provided with the CPA to delivery. The co-ordinator will be responsible for ensuring that an appropriate assessment of the user's health and social care needs is conducted, within a care plan devised and agreed with users and, where appropriate, their carers and co-ordinators.

A copy of the written care plan should be provided to the user and any plan should include contingency plans so that users and or carers can contact specialist services if necessary. It is also contingent on the co-ordinator to provide a copy of the plan to the GP.

Having agreed the care provision necessary the co-ordinator is responsible for ensuring that services are delivered at the right time, in the right environment by appropriately competent community team workers.

Who are the clients?

It is commonly thought that users of mental health services are their clients, yet this only illustrates half the story. Those who use our services have already been identified as either at risk or as suffering from a mental health problem; in addition, the carers of individuals with mental health problems are increasingly seen as clients, and the Carers (Recognition and Services) Act (1995) should be applied to ensure that individual carers have their rights and needs recognized in relation to their caring responsibilities. However, it is worth noting that mental health problems can result from a range of adverse factors, associated with (amongst other things) social exclusion, unemployment, poverty and physical illness (Goldberg and Huxley, 1980; Falloon and Fadden, 1993). All health and social care professionals therefore need to be alert for opportunities to undertake mental health promotion and, where appropriate, to identify risk associated with mental health problems, with their clients. Therefore, all the primary care team, including for example social workers, midwives, health visitors, district nurses and GPs, need to be aware of those factors which may increase the possibility of individuals suffering from mental health problems and to refer those at risk appropriately. The *Mental Health National Service Framework* (DOH, 1999) has reviewed literature extensively and identified common risk factors which are often related to the exacerbation of mental health breakdown (Table 4.3). These may be usefully considered when undertaking a health and social care assessment of individuals or families, even if a mental health issue is not the original reason for referral.

Focus of care

A central focus of community care should be to promote mental health in the community, monitor and stabilize health status and, wherever possible, to improve mental health status and prevent deterioration. Although a detailed approach to assessment using CPA has been described in this chapter, there are many individuals who will receive care associated with mental health problems without requiring standard or enhanced CPA. To illustrate the way in which comprehensive mental health care can be provided to individuals three scenarios are described in the next section of this chapter. All treatment

Table 4.3 Common risk factors which may influence mental health status (DOH, 1999)

Unemployment may be linked to depression
Children in the poorest households are three times more likely to have mental health problems than children in well-off households
Half of all women and a quarter of all men will be affected by depression at some point in their lives
Those who have been abused or have been victims of domestic violence have higher rates of mental health problems
Between a quarter and a half of people using night shelters or sleeping rough may have a serious mental health disorder and up to half of these may be alcohol-dependent
Some Black and ethnic minority groups diagnosed as having higher rates of mental disorder than the general population; refugees are particularly vulnerable
There is a high rate of mental disorder in the prison population
People with drug and alcohol problems have higher rates of other mental health problems
People with physical illness have higher rates of mental health problems

programmes which individuals receive, should be dependent on a sound evidence base (DOH, 1991, 1999). A combination of treatments may be selected from a range including medication, cognitive behaviour therapy, psychosocial intervention, family therapy and brief psychotherapy (Carson and Holloway, 1996; Brooker and Repper, 1998). Whichever treatment is selected on the best evidence available to meet an individual user's needs, the co-ordinator of care will need to engage the user and, where appropriate, significant others, including carers, to provide optimum care (Goldberg and Huxley, 1980; Cox, 1998).

THERAPEUTIC RELATIONSHIPS AND CARE PLANNING

The selection of a model or concepts appropriate to nursing practice are influenced by individual practitioners' beliefs and values, and those associated with the team of which they are a member. Peplau (1952) argues that nursing is essentially an interpersonal process between patient and nurse which should involve a therapeutic focus. The goal of nursing is to assist and educate patients to develop their own ability to cope with problems, anxieties and tensions. Peplau (1952) describes four phases in any such relationship: orientation, identification, exploitation and resolution. The phases are not directly akin to those associated with CPA of assessment, planning, implementation and evaluation but can be applied in a similar manner.

In the *orientation* phase, Peplau (1952) suggests that a nurse may function as a resource providing specific information to help patients to understand their problems; at the same time Peplau (1952) suggests that the beginnings of a counselling relationship may emerge, with the nurse listening to the patient's and/or carer's perception of the problems. Peplau (1952) argues that it is imperative in this phase that the nurse explains to the patient the difficulties of the situation from the nurse's perspective and the types of services that may be available to the patient to assist in resolving problems. Patients also describe their perceptions of their needs and problems. It is the understanding of each other's worlds at this point that is vital to the development of the interpersonal relationship. Clearly, there will be times when both nurse and patient perceptions of any situation are very similar and others when they diverge. When a patient is acutely psychotic, for example, he may describe himself as feeling very well with no problems at all, whereas the nurse perceives a severely distressed individual who is displaying confusion and possibly delusions. In such situations Peplau (1952) would argue that the nurse has to take a lead during that acute illness phase and try to assist the patient to perceive some of the problems that the nurse conceptualizes during assessment or orientation with the patient. The nurse's main aim during the orientation phase is to enable patients to recognize and understand their difficulties and the extent of their need for help.

The second phase of the relationship involves the nurse helping patients to understand the meaning of the situation. Almost inevitably there is an overlap between the orientation and the *identification* stage. Peplau (1952) acknowledges this and argues that the nursing process is a soft system rather than a hard system and cannot follow a linear progression. It may be helpful to think of the orientation and identification phases as a continuum but the third phase, labelled *exploitation*, is clearly a progressive stage from identification. During the exploitation phase the patient accepts the services offered in fulfilment of his interests and needs, hence deriving full value from the relationship. In the majority of cases the exploitation phase is associated with the implementation phase of the nursing process. In Peplau's (1952) model it is expected that patients *assume some responsibility* for their health care at the exploitation phase, no matter how distressed or ill, and are treated very much more as equal partners than is the case in some nurse—patient relationships described by other theorists.

The final and fourth stage of the interpersonal relationship occurs when patients become independent from the nurse and are able to resume full responsibility for their health care. Clearly, the *resolution* stage will be achieved with most patients. Resolution of the immediate situation may be achieved and patients discharged from nursing care; however, in some circumstances, due to the nature of a patient's mental health problems, there is a duty on the nurse to monitor and support patients over prolonged periods. In such circumstances, it is possible for nurse and patient to return to the identification stage of the care process. At this point the nurse can explain the monitoring and supporting role so that patients clearly understand that they are being encouraged to retain their independence in terms of the successful resolution of previous mental health needs. Once both patient and nurse are clear that they accept the jointly agreed plan associated with monitoring and supporting to prevent relapse, the exploitation phases can be re-entered on that understanding. Figure 4.1 illustrates how the phases associated with Peplau's (1952) model can be implemented to care for patients during crisis and ongoing monitoring scenarios.

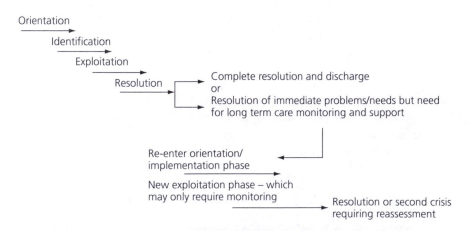

Figure 4.1 A therapeutic model of nursing care (after Peplau, 1952) illustrating the overlap of phases and return to orientation/edentification phase for monitoring and supervision.

Throughout the nurse–patient relationship Peplau (1952) states that the nurse will select appropriate functions and roles according to the patient's needs and requests, and the nurse's knowledge of the situation. She terms these as:

- A resource person.
- A counsellor.
- A surrogate parent.
- A leader.
- A teacher.

The use of the term 'surrogate parent' is unacceptable to some mental health nurses today and many replace this function with that of acting as 'an advocate'. Although the role of advocate is much more common in day-to-day practice, Peplau (1952) describes the function of acting as a 'surrogate parent' in a psychodynamic context; readers may wish to explore this further in the original text if they have a particular interest in psychodynamic intervention. For the majority of community nurses the combined roles of resource person, counsellor, advocate, leader and teacher can be utilized to deliver health promotion, monitoring, education and support to patients with acute and long term mental health problems.

CLIENT-FOCUSED SCENARIOS

Three client scenarios are now presented to illustrate how multi-professional community care teams may work to prevent mental health deterioration and resolve mental health problems in community settings. These scenarios are based on real cases, which have been altered significantly to prevent recognition and maintain confidentiality. They illustrate how selecting a structure for care planning and providing research-based intervention can assist in reaching resolution for users with mental health problems in community settings. Each section for individual scenarios has separate headings to indicate the phase of Peplau's (1952) model that is being utilized at any one time in comparison to the stage of the process associated with CPA.

Case scenario 1 – Anna (involving a community team encompassing a midwife, GP and community mental health nurse)

Assessment/orientation

Anna, a 28-year-old Asian woman married to a Caucasian, was expecting her first baby in three months. When she attended a routine ante-natal appointment the midwife assessed that she was extremely worried about labour. The midwife was particularly concerned because on further enquiry it emerged that a couple of years previously Anna had followed her husband on an overseas appointment and had become severely depressed away from her extended family and friends in England. Her husband had been moved back to England by his firm and there had been no evidence of any further depression subsequent to that return. The picture that emerged as the midwife sympathetically discussed the whole issue of labour with Anna, was of an individual who had left home fairly young but had had a very structured extended family and friendship network. When her husband had moved she had had to give up work and her associated social and family network. The accumulation of those two life events had contributed to the development of a depressive illness. The stress-vulnerability model of mental disorder suggests that it is an accumulation of stress and an associate vulnerability to a mental health illness that often triggers the exacerbation of symptoms (Falloon and Fadden, 1993). The midwife was aware of the stress-vulnerability model and structured her discussion and assessment of Anna appropriately to collect relevant data. She assessed that Anna was concerned that she might suffer a recurrence of depression associated with her fear of the pain of labour, combined with giving up her job for a short period while on maternity leave, and the expectations of having a change in her role associated with motherhood. It materialized that Anna had been unable to discuss any of these fears with her husband.

Formulation of care plan/*orientation* and *identification*

The midwife discussed Anna's case at a clinical supervision session held regularly in the surgery with the GP responsible for ante-natal clinics, the second midwife and the community mental health nurse attached to the clinic. Following discussion, it was agreed that Anna was at high risk of becoming depressed again and it would be necessary to ensure that at her next ante-natal appointment, issues were further discussed and if necessary, Anna referred to the GP. Both the GP and community mental health nurse recommended to the midwife that, if possible, Anna should be encouraged to bring her husband to the ante-natal clinic at the next visit to see whether an opportunity could be used to discuss Anna's fears with her husband. Her husband had reportedly been very supportive when she had been depressed before and was likely to be so again.

Intervention/*exploitation* involving clients

The midwife telephoned Anna to see how she was doing and Anna said that she had felt much better for discussing the situation with the midwife but had not as yet discussed her fears with her husband. The midwife suggested to Anna that it might be helpful to bring her husband to the next ante-natal clinic where some of Anna's concerns could be aired between the three of them. Anna said that although she thought this would be helpful, she could not see why her husband should think it necessary to come to the clinic. The midwife suggested that one way for Anna to encourage her husband to attend the clinic would be to point out to him that he would be able to hear the baby's heartbeat during the ante-natal session if he wanted to do so. Anna thought he would be very keen to do this. At the next ante-natal clinic Anna attended with her husband, Jim.

Jim was excited to hear the baby's heartbeat and the midwife was able to explain that although hearing the heartbeat was very exciting, it also brought the birth of the baby nearer and asked whether he had any concerns about the birth of the baby. Jim said that his main concern was for Anna and, in particular, whether she was nervous about the situation; he knew that he was sometimes quite difficult to talk to and he had not raised this with Anna himself. The three then discussed at length some of Anna's fears, in particular concerning giving up work a month before the baby was due and the subsequent loss of friendships associated with work. Jim pointed out that he was going to take some leave, both prior to the baby being born and immediately afterwards, and that he would be very happy if Anna wanted to go and stay with her elder sister for a couple of weeks leading up to the birth, as she lived only 30 miles away.

At this point, Anna was able to express her own fears, in particular, that she might become depressed again. She reiterated the concerns she had in relation to labour, giving up her job and the responsibilities of having to care for a baby 24 hours a day. Jim was extremely reassuring, pointing out that she had responded very well to cognitive therapy when she had been ill before and she had not needed any medication. Anna then explained that she would not wish to take any medication because she wanted to breastfeed. The midwife confirmed that as Anna had responded very well to cognitive therapy in the past, medication was unlikely to be necessary, even if she did become depressed again. The midwife was then able to ask Anna whether she would like to see the community mental health nurse for some brief cognitive therapy to discuss some of her fears about the birth and the change to her lifestyle. Anna said that she thought that this would be very helpful, as a community mental health nurse had been very supportive to her in the past.

Cognitive approach to intervention/*exploitation*
The community mental health nurse saw Anna every two weeks before the birth of her baby, using a cognitive approach to treatment and encouraging Anna to develop her ability to discuss her fears with Jim and to keep her social networks up during the month immediately prior to the birth. Anna attended regularly and was committed to the partnership of trying to overcome her anxieties. She had a copy of her care plan and was able to refer to this as necessary during this period.

Anna proceeded to have her baby and did suffer moderate post-natal depression. She was successfully treated with cognitive therapy and supportive intervention from family and friends. Jim needed considerable support early on and learned to support Anna by reducing her stress associated with loss of work friends, by agreeing to her returning to work earlier than originally anticipated. An excellent day nursery was found for their baby and Anna returned to work two days a week, four months after the baby was born.

Resolution
Within a year Anna felt able to suggest that she stopped seeing the community mental health nurse as she felt well and no longer at risk of suffering a relapse of depression. She felt very positive about the way in which she had developed her role as a mother and was thoroughly enjoying taking care of

her baby, sharing responsibilities within the extended family and working part-time. She continued to say that she had found labour difficult and quite frightening, but felt reassured that if she had a second baby she had successfully got through what for her had been a stressful situation. The community mental health nurse concurred with Anna's self-assessment and discharged her from active management while reinforcing that Anna was free to contact her again if she felt further help may be of assistance or to telephone NHS Direct for help and advice at any time.

Summary

This scenario describes an example of teamwork within a general practice setting with a midwife using a routine ante-natal assessment to identify risk factors associated with depression. This enabled early preventative treatment to be undertaken prior to the user displaying frank systems of depression. This meant that early cognitive therapy intervention was conducted and although Anna suffered some post-natal depression, the relationship between her, the midwife and the community mental health nurse had already developed sufficiently resulting in successful support and treatment post-natally. The family's response to Anna's depression was good with Jim being supportive and agreeing to a change in the plans that had originally been set for Anna to have a year off work after her first baby. The family and social network that was available to Anna was extremely supportive and this was partly because the depressive illness did not become severe owing partly to early intervention and appropriate treatment. It is well-recognized that where families can be supportive with individuals who suffer a mental health problem, sufferers are more likely to regain independence and mental health, than where families have not been involved in understanding the care provision (Mental Health Foundation, 2000).

Case scenario 2 – James (involving a community team comprising a GP, consultant psychiatrist, social worker, health visitor and community mental health nurse)

Assessment/*orientation*

A community mental health nurse was asked by the GP to visit James. The following information was passed over.

James was a 32-year-old man with a history of severe enduring mental illness. He had been at university for two years when he was first diagnosed as having a schizophrenic illness. Following his second year exams at university he had had a psychotic breakdown and had been unable to return to university the following year. He had been successfully treated as an inpatient, during his acute psychotic stage, with appropriate medication and stabilized on phenothiazines. He had returned to university, graduated and begun work as a senior administrative assistant in a telecommunications firm. He had attended his local surgery regularly for medication and had not had a relapse for nearly ten years.

James was married, aged 28, to a secretary who was well aware of his illness and the fact that he was on long-term medication. His wife, Jane, was reserved, relatively emotionally undemanding and very supportive of James. She was also proud of his seniority at work and believed that he should seek promotion.

Approximately six weeks before the assessment James and his wife had a baby girl, Janet. James had found taking on a father's role quite difficult, particularly when he was kept awake at night by the baby. The GP had been to visit the family following Jane coming to a routine post-natal visit with her baby. Jane had broken down at that visit and said that she was having great difficulty keeping the child quiet at night and that James had actually shouted at both her and the baby, although he had never shouted at her before.

It was decided that the GP and community mental health nurse would do a joint assessment visit to the home. Access to the home was relatively easy in that Jane welcomed them in and James was home from work. It was immediately evident that James was becoming increasingly irritable and short-tempered with both his wife and baby. Some discussion ensued and James explained that he could not go to work because he was so exhausted from the baby keeping him awake at night and other issues. The GP asked for clarification on other issues. James said, 'Well, you know there's so many people keeping me awake at night and generally I'm exhausted because, [pause] well, I just keep eating and I've put on weight, and as you know I'm just working so hard at work and Jane doesn't go to work anymore because of the baby, and I'm having to be much more careful with money, and anyway at night I just can't sleep properly'.

It was quite clear that James was stressed and that the changing life events associated with his wife giving up work, the birth of his baby and broken nights associated with parenthood, were beginning to result in James displaying symptoms associated with a possible recurrence of an acute schizophrenia episode (Falloon and Fadden, 1993). Recognizing that specialist mental health service intervention may be necessary, the community mental health nurse and the GP asked James whether he would be willing to see the consultant psychiatrist. James agreed to do this, albeit reluctantly, but said to the psychiatrist, 'I will for my family and also to get everything sorted out, and perhaps you would like to find a way of keeping the child quiet at night.' The second part of this remark alerted the team to further concerns that James's main concern was to keep the child quiet at night, rather than having any insight into his own unreasonable expectation that such a small baby would sleep all through the night. It was clear that James thought the best way of coping would be to get 'back to normal' and lead a more regulated existence. The lack of insight into some of the problem being his own difficulty with coping was an indication that he might be losing touch with reality (Goldberg and Huxley, 1980) in that his new baby could not be expected to conform to an adult lifestyle.

The consultant psychiatrist assessed James in outpatients and said that he, too, was concerned about James's potential for suffering a mental health crisis. He suggested that James have a slight increase in medication and that there be a multi-professional case conference to discuss James's immediate care needs.

The community mental health nurse discussed the situation with the family's health visitor, who arranged to visit Jane and offer any appropriate support for her in relation to caring for the baby.

Planning care/*identification* – multi-professional case conference/*identification*

The health visitor and social worker were asked to the case conference, in particular to consider the potential risks to the child associated with James's illness. After very careful consideration, the multi-professional team decided that it would attempt to provide assertive outreach support (Knapp *et al.*, 1994; Burns and Santes, 1995; Onyett, 1995) to James and his family, to try and reduce the tension within the family and prevent the need for an inpatient episode for him. The health visitor suggested that she increase her observational and supportive visits to the family to twice a week with the focus of her role being on ensuring the baby was receiving appropriate care. This action was agreed.

James and Jane were seen together and the psychiatrist and community mental health nurse explained that they were worried that there was a possibility of James having a relapse and, in particular, that his tiredness and exhaustion might result in him becoming increasingly irritable with the family. Jane explained that while she was very happy not to make demands on James during this difficult period, she could not guarantee that the baby would not wake them in the night. The care plan, a copy of which was given to James, focused on using increased medication and a psychosocial intervention (Mari *et al.*, 1996; Fadden, 1998) approach to try to reduce the stress associated with changing family dynamics. A structured approach to a care plan was agreed and James felt that it would be wise for him to have a period off work for two weeks to see whether, by reducing the demands of work, he felt more able to cope at home.

Implementation/*exploitation*

During that two weeks the community mental health nurse visited on a daily basis to continue to assess the situation and to work with James to ensure that he was taking medication and to discuss some of the issues associated with the change in his life. James was able to express his pleasure at having a new daughter during these visits, but also his concerns relating to the change to his routine. The health visitor continued to visit and felt that Jane and James were providing appropriate parental care of their baby, even though Jane was carrying the majority of the care.

The community mental health nurse used the principles of psychosocial intervention with Jane, explaining that during this period where James was bordering on a psychotic episode, it was very important to try and reduce demands on him and to ensure that he slept regularly (Goldberg and Huxley, 1980; Fadden, 1998). At the same time the nurse discussed how Jane was feeling and acknowledged the stress associated with supporting James. The nurse assessed that Jane was well able to cope at that point by using an appropriate structure for the assessment of caregiver burden (Schene *et al.*, 1994). James agreed to take some night sedation and at the end of two weeks' structured intervention, was sleeping regularly, although Jane was rather tired getting up to the baby by herself. At a joint health visitor and community mental health nurse meeting Jane said that though she was tired this was much less stressful than when she was worried about James and the baby. James could see that he would need to continue to take the slightly increased anti-psychotic medication for a period and also his night medication to sleep through the night. It was agreed that Jane's mother would come and stay for three or four nights and help her with the baby during the night, to give her a bit of a break and that James would go and stay for the weekend with his mother who was well able to provide him with a period of quiet and rest. This occurred and when James returned home after the weekend, Jane had had a good rest and was feeling much better; she had enjoyed being cared for by her mother. James also had appreciated going home to his mother and realizing how much he missed Jane and the baby.

Resolution of crisis

Although both Jane and James were well aware that in the long term James may become ill again and may at some point need inpatient admission, they were both proud that they had got through a relatively difficult patch without that being necessary. Jane became much more used to the baby and found herself more able to structure her day so that she was less demanding on James when he returned from work at night. The principles here of psychosocial intervention, particularly with Jane, and explaining the illness and the illness pattern to her in the structure of the vulnerability-stress model (Falloon and Fadden, 1993) enabled her to support James during this period. James's commitment to his marriage and the small amount of insight he had into his illness allowed him to take some responsibility for his own mental health care and his willingness to take increased medication and night sedation certainly contributed to his reaching mental health stability much more quickly than would have been achieved otherwise.

Return to implementation phase

Due to the nature of James's health care problems, it would be necessary for the team to continue to monitor and support James on a long-term basis in line with CPA. Peplau (1952) would suggest that the key worker should re-enter the orientation phase with James to undertake an identification of future goals to plan for future long-term care intervention associated with a new exploitation phase.

Scenario 3 – Hugh and Joyce (involving a care team including a community mental health nurse, GP, speech therapist, practice nurse, district nurse, physiotherapist and inpatient and day patient health care staff)

Assessment/*orientation* and *identification*

Joyce and Hugh had been married for 47 years; neither had had any mental ill health until Hugh had a cerebral vascular accident that resulted in him being left with severe short-term memory loss, confusion and irritability. He also ceased to show normal emotion and, although recognizing his wife, was unsympathetic to any of her needs.

Joyce had been very shocked when Hugh had collapsed when they had been out shopping and had worked extremely hard during the six weeks he was in hospital to try and encourage his rehabilitation. Immediately after Hugh's stroke it had been explained to her that he should make progress in the next two to three months and after that would probably be relatively stable. Joyce had really focused on Hugh's physical problems; when first in hospital he was unable to feed himself, walk or look after his own elimination needs. Gradually with structured physiotherapy in hospital, he began to walk with a stick, was able to take himself to the toilet, wash and dress, although all these activities were relatively slow. Once or twice while he was in hospital he had become very irritated. Joyce reported that when she had asked him a question he had actually sworn at her for the first time in her life. On discharge home Hugh was provided with speech therapy, physiotherapy and district nursing support. After two visits the district nurse explained that she would not be coming any more as Joyce was able to assist Hugh with his daily living needs, he was speaking relatively well, mostly able to make himself understood and sleeping regularly. He was not at risk of developing pressure sores as he was able to walk around their very comfortable flat and appeared to be physically well. The district nurse explained that Hugh should attend the practice nurse at least once a week to have his blood pressure monitored and that this weekly visit should reduce over time once this was more stable. Joyce was quite happy about this as Joyce and Hugh were relatively well-off and it was quite easy for them to take a taxi to visit the practice nurse.

After four visits, the physiotherapist explained that Hugh was now able to walk freely around the flat with his stick, use the lift downstairs and get up and down four or five steps which was really all he needed to be able to do in terms of managing effectively at home. She therefore discontinued her visits. The speech therapist discharged Hugh from her books but did write to the GP saying that though there was no more that she could do to assist Hugh, his speech was such that he could be understood by Joyce but that at times he did appear still to get confused when he was tired and was sometimes very irritable with Joyce. The speech therapist visited for nearly a month and was very supportive to Joyce and understood that sometimes Hugh was very irritable with her.

Joyce arrived for a routine visit with the practice nurse to have Hugh's blood pressure taken, with a nasty bruise on her face. The practice nurse said, 'What have you been doing to your face, Joyce?' at which Hugh immediately said, 'She walked into a door, she's such a silly old cow.'; the practice nurse was very surprised as she had never heard him swear like this before. She said, 'Are you alright Hugh?' Hugh said, 'Who would bloody be all right with such a silly old cow; I've had enough I don't want to live with her any more.'; at this Joyce looked down at her clothes and very quietly started to cry with tears pouring down her cheeks. The practice nurse realized that there was a very difficult situation and asked Hugh to wait outside while she talked to his wife. He picked up his stick and poked the practice nurse with it, saying, *'I will bloody stay here if I want to!'* The practice nurse moved towards the door, called the receptionist and asked her to summon the GP. The GP came out of his office and at this Hugh stood up and started to shout almost incomprehensibly, became very red in the face and then suddenly half collapsed back into his chair. Hugh was irritable and confused, possibly associated with his cerebral vascular accident. It was quite clear that a crisis was emerging between Joyce and Hugh. After some discussion it was agreed that Hugh would be admitted to hospital for further assessment and Joyce would go home in a taxi, with the GP arranging to visit her later that afternoon.

Plan and implementation/*identification* and *exploitation*

The GP went to visit Joyce with a community mental health nurse who had a special interest in supporting older people at home, and discovered that Joyce was bruised in several places. Joyce acknowledged that Hugh had started to whack her with his walking stick when she did not do as he asked. She was extremely ashamed and could not associate the husband, with whom she had lived so long, with any kind of violence. It materialized that Joyce had lost nearly half a stone in the preceding couple of weeks, that she was having difficulty sleeping, and that she was showing preliminary signs of depression. The GP and community mental health nurse explained that it may be necessary for Hugh to be in some respite care or a nursing home for a short period to establish how psychologically affected he was as a result of his stroke and whether anything could be done to reduce these aggressive outbursts. Joyce explained that she felt that she was failing, that as a wife she should be able to look after her husband until he died in comfort in their home. She explained that she would be happy to pay for somebody to come and sit with him for a period, so she could get out during the day. It was agreed that the community mental health nurse would arrange to see Joyce the following afternoon.

The community mental health nurse visited Joyce and agreed that Joyce should encourage Hugh to come home if she felt this was most appropriate because no overt physical problems had been identified during Hugh's hospital admission that could have contributed to his outbursts. Joyce was very keen to have Hugh home and expressed her willingness to work closely with the community mental health nurse to try and manage the difficult situation. The community mental health nurse agreed a care plan with Joyce that focused on her trying to meet Hugh's needs when he first demanded attention, but also enabling Joyce to express her needs to Hugh. In particular, she was encouraged to express the fact that she could not accept being hit again and that if violence continued to occur, it would be necessary either to have additional support at home or for Joyce to consider Hugh being admitted to a nursing home. It was agreed that Joyce would not discuss these issues immediately with Hugh on his return home, but rather that over a series of constructive one-hour sessions between the community mental health nurse, Joyce and Hugh, these issues would be explored. Both Joyce and Hugh agreed independent care plans to meet their own needs with the community mental health nurse. They kept copies of these care plans to refer to; Joyce's involved taking more control over her situation based on a cognitive model of intervention (Beck *et al.*, 1987).

Implementation/*exploitation*

During the next six weeks the community mental health nurse visited Joyce and Hugh three times a week; discussion took place as to why Hugh felt frustrated with his disablement and additional speech therapy was organized in an attempt to assist Hugh to overcome his frustration associated with speech difficulties. In order to give Joyce a break these sessions were arranged at a local day hospital and Hugh agreed to visit the day hospital two full days a week. This enabled Joyce to undertake her routine household tasks while Hugh was at the day hospital and gave her more time to focus on his needs and be with him when he was at home.

No further episodes of physical violence were reported by Joyce and she began to express clearly some of her own needs to Hugh in the sessions led by the community mental health nurse. In particular, she expressed her need to get out and about with Hugh and to try and resume some of their social life despite his frustration in relation to his speech. They began to go out regularly once a week to an activity that did not include the need for talking. Visiting the cinema, going shopping and having a cup of coffee were both activities that Joyce enjoyed and that Hugh was able to undertake without becoming too frustrated; indeed, he said he quite enjoyed going to the cinema. Joyce was clear that in the event of Hugh ever becoming physically violent again, she would have to discuss this with the GP and community mental health nurse, whereas Hugh was very distressed that he had actually ever been violent. In fact, he denied being able to remember it, but was able to remember being very angry with Joyce. She explained that she could accept him occasionally shouting as he had always done this during their marriage but that physical violence was unacceptable.

Evaluation/*resolution*

At the end of six weeks Joyce felt much happier with caring for Hugh but continued to be anxious about their future. She had not been treated with any drugs for her depression but had learned, through the structured cognitive approach selected by the nurse, to cope with some of the increasing demands made on her as a full time carer. During the period described, Hugh had regained some independence and was much happier going out into the garden and had even begun to read and use his music centre more independently than he had before the crisis had emerged in the GP's surgery. Until that point, Joyce said Hugh had adopted a very dependent role and had not actually been making an effort to do some things that he could. It was agreed that the community mental health nurse would visit once a month for the next three months to continue to monitor the situation, but after the intensive six-week intervention, she felt it appropriate to discharge Joyce and Hugh from her books with the exception of the monitoring sessions. She left appropriate telephone numbers of local services and NHS Direct for Joyce to contact in the event of a crisis.

Summary

This scenario indicates that supporting a partner after a stroke can result in a carer developing mental health problems associated with significant caring responsibilities and change in the partner's behaviour. A brief cognitive therapy approach to this situation enhanced the lives of both carer and the person receiving care. There was a danger at the beginning of this crisis that Joyce (the carer) would become a user of the mental health services over a prolonged period but satisfactory resolution did occur relatively swiftly, associated with comprehensive health care intervention. The improvement in Hugh's state was partially attributable to Joyce taking some control over the situation and being encouraged to express her own needs, and expecting Hugh to accept more responsibility for his own health and behaviour than she had done on his initial discharge from hospital.

Consider the following questions in relation to the three case scenarios:

- Consider the criteria that would inform the team in making a decision regarding CPA for each client? Table 4.2 may assist you in this work.
- Did any of the users require formal CPA?
- If so, would CPA have been defined as standard or enhanced?
- Which professional involved in each scenario do you think emerged as the key worker for the period of care described? Discuss the rationale for your conclusions with another colleague and see if they agree.
- Which if either of the two primary care standards as defined in the NHS framework for mental health do you think applied in each scenario? Were they wholly or partially met? Consider the criteria in Table 4.1.
- To what extent do you believe the criteria identified in the section on the NHS framework for mental health in relation to the services people with mental health problems can expect to receive, were achieved in each scenario? Try to grade this on a scale of one to five using 'Effectively achieved' (5) 'Not achieved at all' (1). In some instances it may be necessary to discard the criteria as not applicable because of the insufficient information in the scenario but try not to exclude evaluating the extent to which they were achieved for any other reason.
- Which, if any, of the functions described by Peplau (1952) (using advocacy as a substitute for 'surrogate parent'), were adopted by health workers in each scenario?
- To what extent were interventions evidence-based in each scenario?
- Finally, identify at lease three methods by which you could have enhanced the care described. For example, could referral to a user support group have helped in the care provision?

Conclusion

This chapter has outlined some of the issues associated with providing community care to individuals with mental health problems. It illustrates that there is a need to provide a specified range of services for users, their families, friends and informal carers. The newly developed *Mental Health National Service Framework* (DOH, 1999) gives clear specifications for services that are to be provided for individuals in both health and social care settings to meet the targets identified. The chapter has focused primarily on delivering care to individuals, the most common role of community mental health nurses. It must be noted, however, that roles may change as assertive outreach teams and crisis intervention services develop over the next five years to meet the targets required of the NHS framework. It will be important to evaluate the effects of developing services on users and carers and to find out whether 24-hour home treatment teams will become the norm throughout the UK (Holloway, 1997; Mingella, 1998; Perkins and Repper, 1998). It is quite clear that, wherever possible, clients wish to be cared for in community settings and that provided sufficient community resources are made available, the majority may be able to avoid inpatient admission. If individuals are to be monitored and supervised at home while being assessed as at risk to themselves or others, careful consideration will have to be given to the provision of safe effective services. This chapter has not attempted to describe how such supervision may be provided, partly because new legislation will need to be enacted if clients are to be contained outside a hospital structure. It is clear, however, that there are significant challenges ahead for community mental health teams as comprehensive supportive services for individuals and their families are increasingly provided in community health and social care settings.

References

Beck, A., Rush, A.K.J., Shaw, B.F. and Emery, G. (1979) *Cognitive therapy of depression.* New York: Guildford Press.

Brooker, C. and Repper, J. (eds) (1998) *Serious mental health problems in the community: policy, practice and research.* London: Balliere Tindall.

Burns, B.J. and Santos, A.B. (1995) Assertive community treatment: an update of randomised trials. *Psychiatric Services*, 46: 669–73.

Campbell, P. (1989) Peter Campbell's story. In: Brackx, A. and Grimshaw, C. (eds) *Mental health care in crisis.* London: Pluto.

Caplin, R.D., Proudfoot, J., Guest, D. and Carson, J. (1997) Effect of cognitive–behavioural training on job-finding among long term unemployed people. *Lancet* 350, 96.

Carson, J. and Holloway, F. (1996) Interventions with long term clients. In: Watkins, M., Hervey, N., Carson, J. and Ritter, S. (eds) *Collaborative community mental health care.* London: Arnold.

Cox, A. (1998) User centred mental health assessments. *The Mental Health Review*, 3: 2.

Department of Health. (1991) *Report for health: an R&D strategy for the NHS*. London: HMSO (Sir Michael Peckham, Chairman).

Department of Health. (1994) *Implementing caring for people: care management*. London: HMSO.

Department of Health. (1995) *Building bridges: a guide to arrangements for inter-agency working for the care and protection of severely mentally ill people*. London: HMSO.

Department of Health for England. (1999) *Mental health national service frameworks*. London: DOH.

Fadden, G. (1998) Family intervention. In: Brooker, C. and Repper, J. (eds) *Serious mental health problems in the community: policy, practice and research*. London: Bailliere Tindall; 159–83.

Falloon, I. and Fadden, G. (1993) *Integrated mental health care. A comprehensive community based approach*. Cambridge: Cambridge University Press.

Goldberg, D. and Huxley, P. (1980) *Mental illness in the community. The pathway to psychiatric care*. London: Tavistock Publications.

Hervey, N., Carson, J. and Ritter, S. (1996) *Collaborative community mental health care*. London: Edward Arnold.

Holloway, F. (1997) 24 hour nursed care for people with severe and enduring mental illness. *Psychiatric Bulletin*, 21: 195–6.

Kagan, N., Kagan, H. and Watson, M. (1992) Stress reduction in the workplace: the effectiveness of psychoeducational programmes. *Journal of Counselling Psychology*, 42: 71–8.

Kemp, R., Kirov, G., Everitt, B. and David A (1998) A randomised controlled trial of compliance therapy: 18 month follow-up. *British Journal of Psychiatry*, 172: 413–19.

Knapp, M., Beecham, J., Koutsogeorgopoulou, V. *et al.* (1994) Services use and costs of home-based versus hospital-based care for people with serious mental illness. *British Journal of Psychiatry*, 165: 195–203.

Lucas, J. (1996) Multidisciplinary care in the community for clients with mental health problems: guidelines for the future. In: Watkins, M., Hervey, N., Carson, J. and Ritter, S. (eds) *Collaborative community mental health care*. London: Arnold; 350–71.

Mari, J., Adams, C. and Streiner, D. (1996). *Family intervention for those with schizophrenia*. The Cochrane Library: BMJ Publications (most recent amendment 23 February 1996).

Mental Health Foundation. (1997) *Knowing our own minds: a survey of how people in emotional distress take control of their lives*. London: Mental Health Foundation.

Mental Health Foundation. (1999) *Bright futures – promoting children and young people's mental health*. London: Mental Health Foundation.

Mental Health Foundation. (2000) *Pull yourself together! A survey of people's experience of stigma and discrimination as a result of mental distress*. London: Mental Health Foundation.

MIND. (1983) *Common concerns: MIND's manifesto*. London: MIND.

MIND. (1993a) Policy on black and minority ethnic people and mental health. In: *MINDfile 1 Policy*. London: MIND.

MIND. (1993b) *Breakthrough: making community care work. MIND campaign pack*. London: MIND.

Minghella, E. *et al.* (1998) *Open all hours: a model of 24 hour response for people with mental health emergencies*. London: Sainsbury Centre for Mental Health.

Morgan, S. (1998) The assessment and management of risk. In: Brooker, C. and Repper,

J. (eds) *Serious mental health problems in the community: policy, practice and research.* London: Bailliere Tindall; 264–90.

NHS Centre for Reviews and Dissemination. (1997) Mental health promotion in high risk groups. *Effective Health Care Bulletin,* 3.

NHS Centre for Reviews and Dissemination. (1999) Drug treatments for schizophrenia. *Effective Health Care Bulletin,* 5.

Onyett, S.R. (1995) Responsibility and accountability in community mental health teams. *Psychiatric Bulletin,* 19: 281–5.

Peck, E. (1998) Purchasing mental health services. In: Brooker, C. and Repper, J. (eds) *Serious mental health problems in the community: policy, practice and research.* London: Bailliere Tindall; 36–61.

Peplau, H. (1952) *Interpersonal relations in nursing.* New York: G.P. Putnam.

Perkins, R.E. and Repper, J. (1998) Principles of working with people who experience mental health problems. In: Brooker, C. and Repper, J. (eds) *Serious mental health problems in the community: policy, practice and research.* London: Bailliere Tindall; 14–35.

Ritchie, J., Dick, D. and Lingham, R. (1994) *The report of the committee of inquiry into the care and support of Christopher Clunis.* London: HMSO.

Schene, A.H., Tessler, R.C. and Gamache, G.M. (1994) Instruments measuring family of caregiver burden in severe mental illness. *Social Psychiatry and Psychiatric Epidemiology,* 29: 229–40.

Social Service Inspectorate and NHS Executive. (1996) *Effective care co-ordination in mental health services: modernising the care programme approach – a policy booklet.* London: DOH.

Somerset Health Authority and Somerset Social Services. (2000) *Report of the independent inquiry into the care and treatment of Ms Justine Cummings.* (Lord Laming, Chairman).

Strathdee, G. and Sutherby, K. (1996) Liaison psychiatry and primary health care settings. In: Watkins, M., Hervey, N., Carson, J. and Ritter, S. (eds) *Collaborative community mental health care.* London: Arnold.

Further reading and bibliography

Department of Health. (1997) *Modernising mental health services: safe, sound, secure.* London: HMSO.

Department of Health and the Welsh Office. (1999) Mental Health Act 1983: Code of Practice London: The Stationery Office.

Knudsen, H.E. and Thorncroft, G. (eds) (1996) *Mental health service evaluation.* Cambridge: Cambridge University Press.

Mari, J.J. and Streiner, D. (1996) *Family intervention for people with schizophrenia.* Cochrane Review: Oxford Update Software, Oxford.

Family caregivers and community nurses: co-experts in care?

Lorly McClure

Introduction

Over the last decade, the pivotal role of informal, lay or family caregivers has been legitimized within British social policy. Service providers have been exhorted to make practical support for informal carers a priority (DOH, 1990, 1997). Informal carers have been given 'the right to an assessment of their own needs (DOH, 1996) and the British government has introduced, and promised funding for, a new policy package, outlined in *Caring for Carers, A National Strategy for Carers* (DOH, 1999).

This new-found prominence of informal carers in the UK is the consequence of a range of social developments this century. The efficacy of modern biomedicine in the Western world, leading to the cure and control of disease, has generated an extensive need and demand for long-term care of chronically sick and disabled people of all ages, especially for those who are frail and elderly (Arber and Ginn, 1990a). Demographic trends indicate a steady increase in the numbers of disabled elderly people likely to be dependent on expensive health and social services (Nolan *et al.*, 1996). Similarly, there has been the spiralling cost of long-term professional care for children and adults with learning or physical disabilities and mental illness. These cost implications have been accompanied by the anticipated reduction in the numbers of women available to provide free care, as well as an acute decline in the recruitment of nurses (DOH, 1999a).

The community care White Paper, *Caring for People* (DOH, 1989), identified the responsibility of local authority social services and the then district health authorities to provide care for elderly, sick and disabled people. However, it was made clear that the greater part of care for these people has been and always will be provided by families and friends, the expectation being that this will persist. Caring in the community therefore continues to be translated into caring by the community (DHSS, 1981), 90% of this care being provided by family members (DOH, 1999).

In the UK, it has recently been estimated that there are 5.7 million people, 3.3 million women and 2.4 million men, who consider themselves to be providing care for a sick, handicapped or elderly person. This indicates that there could be a caregiver in one out of every six households in the country (ONS, 1998). The value originally placed on the contributions which unpaid carers make to 'community care', was calculated at between £15 and £20 billion each year (Family Policy Bulletin, 1989). More recently, according to the Institute of Actuaries in 1993, the expectation is that caregivers will continue to save the British taxpayer an estimated £33 billion a year (Nuttall, 1992).

Given these figures, it is not surprising that, for almost 40 years, British social policy has had a commitment that people who are sick or disabled should be cared for within the community (Parker, 1990). If this estimated £33 billion saving is accurate, the government proposal of allocating an extra £140 million for carers over a three-year period (DOH, 1999) has the potential of being money very well spent. However, disability researchers have expressed concern that the needs of caregivers could be given priority at the expense of those needing care. This could lead to the exploitation of both groups unless the needs of both are adequately addressed (Morris, 1993; Kirk and Glendinning, 1998).

The term 'informal carer' has been in use only since the late 1970s, as hitherto the hidden and unrecognized caring role of women was brought to the fore by feminist writers (Arber and Ginn, 1990b). Within the present chapter, informal carers will be referred to as 'family caregivers' for three reasons. First, experience indicates that carers do not like the term 'informal carer' (Nolan et al., 1996). Second, most 'informal' caring is delivered by family members (DOH, 1999a) and, third, the term 'carer' can be confused with paid carers working in the community, hospitals and voluntary organizations.

Although family caregivers who receive help from the community nursing services are frequently appreciative and full of praise of this, significant limitations are still being identified (Henwood, 1998; Brown and Stetz, 1999). Studies which focus on the needs of caregivers suggest that community nurses tend to direct their attention towards patients, family carers being taken for granted and their needs neglected. This reflects persistent traditional priorities of nursing practice which, in line with Western ideology, has been inclined to focus on the primacy of the individual (Lister, 1997). That aspect of the environment which can include caring family members is not always considered to be a target for nursing intervention (Richardson, 1998).

Kirk and Glendinning (1998) recently refer to two key policy trends that are creating a shift in the boundaries between informal family caregiving and formal community nursing. These are the move from institutional to home care, and the growing development in nursing towards a commitment to partnership and patient participation. The latter is echoed by one of the key initiatives proposed in the recent White Paper, Saving Lives (DOH, 1999b), which proposes an 'expert patients programme' intended to influence the services to those with chronic disease. When considering how community nurses might respond to these changes, this chapter focuses on the experiences of some carers and issues concerning gender, age and ethnicity are examined within specific caring relationships. A discussion about the perceptions that community nurses might have of family caregivers follows and the implications associated with the prospect of family caregivers and community nurses entering into a reciprocal and equal relationship as co-experts in care can then be explored (Nolan *et al.*, 1999).

The caregiving experience

There are as many types of caregivers as there are people in the community, and they can be categorized in many different ways. However, caregiving is embedded in a range of social relationships with family, friends and neighbours which reflect various caring roles and responsibilities.

Here, caring experiences within three significant relationships that prevail in the kinship structure of British society, namely partners, parents and offspring, are considered. Evidence of these caring relationships can frequently be seen by community nurses in their day-to-day practice, as they visit hospitals and work in homes, clinics, surgeries, schools and health centres.

PARTNERS CARING FOR ONE ANOTHER

When disability strikes one or other partners within a relationship, the experiences of the carer can reflect the gender role expectations of society. A woman's caring role may become an extension of her role as a wife, and can be taken for granted by all concerned (Parker, 1993).

> A very frequent comment heard from wives in this situation is that 'I was never asked if I'd be able to manage.' This seems to encapsulate the attitude of professionals: the assumption that the ability to cope is bestowed with the wedding ring. (Judith Oliver who cares for her tetraplegic husband, in Hicks, 1988: 79)

A well-documented difference between the caring experiences of men and women is that men who care are more likely to receive help from statutory agencies (Hicks, 1988). One example is that domestic help will be accepted by male carers as a replacement for the domestic service that their wives are no longer able to provide. However, this help is often forthcoming only after a hard fight, men often being more likely than women to employ forceful tactics to get what they need. Women see domestic work as their responsibility and appear less likely to demand help as long as they are physically able to cope.

Turning to the provision of intimate personal care, it has been assumed that this is not a problem for carers within a marriage or marriage-like relationship (Parker, 1993). This highlights the difference between hospital and home experience. Hospitals are total environments, within which the medical model tends to prevail. On entering hospital, an individual is transformed from a social body to a medical body. High-tech equipment, unfamiliar and often incomprehensible language spoken by a confusing range of uniformed staff, convey symbols which serve to re-negotiate socially accepted rules of privacy and intimacy into a form of neutrality. The social taboos associated with personal care, characterized by touching, nakedness and excreta are overcome. There is an expectation that nurses will do for their patients that which patients cannot do for themselves (Twigg, 1992). Relatives and friends can telephone and visit the hospital, but traditionally, except in the case of young children, hospital nurses usually will protect the privacy of their patients by sending relatives, including spouse or partner, 'out of the room' during intimate nursing procedures (Lawler, 1991).

However, when someone is discharged from hospital with a long-term chronic illness or disability, those relatives often find that their normal social role is extended into many different demanding activities. These can range from additional shopping, cooking, housework, gardening and household repairs, to personal tasks such as washing, dressing, feeding, giving medication, toileting, dealing with incontinence and assisting with mobility.

Parker (1993) who interviewed 22 married couples aged under 65, found that both disabled wives and husbands could be distressed and embarrassed by the nature of care they needed from their partners, such as helping to secure sanitary pads, or coping with incontinence. Nearly all of the couples in this study found that their sexual relationships had been affected in some way. Both carers and cared-for found the need to adapt to a change in their lives together (Parker, 1993).

Ahmad and Atkin (1996) identified a need for in-depth research into the experiences of the 'largely invisible' carers from different ethnic minority groups. In order to enable a more targeted approach to service provision for these caregivers, it is intended that data about ethnic minority caregivers will be collected in the 2001 Census (DOH, 1999). Hicks (1988) suggested that exile, unemployment and poverty experienced by men who are recent immigrants to the UK from the Asian subcontinent has, in many cases, led to chronic physical and mental illness. The expectation from their own ethnic group, as well as from their host society, is that their wives will become their carers – despite speaking little English and with minimal access to social support. This role is frequently undertaken without help either from extended family or from an unfamiliar society and an indifferent health service which fails to understand the family's cultural needs (Hicks, 1988).

Elderly people, whatever their ethnic origin, gender or status, are generally assumed to represent a burden, or potential burden, upon younger relatives, the 'community' and the state. However, it has been shown that older people who need care and are married, are much more likely to be looked after by their partner than by anyone else (DOH, 1999a).

Caring is normally founded on close relationships (DOH, 1999a) and, although caring for a partner might appear to be an onerous burden for an elderly person in poor health, it should not be overlooked that caregiving can also afford a sense of pride, joy and satisfaction (Nolan et al., 1996).

The nature of personal care and domestic work that elderly married men and women undertake within the private domain could be said to be a taken-for-granted obligation of spouse to spouse. This represents a provision of 23%

and 24% of the total hours of co-resident care provided by men and women, respectively, and yet this significant contribution remains hidden and difficult to capture in quantitative surveys (Arber and Ginn, 1990a).

Gender differences have been identified by men and women themselves when discussing their reasons for continuing to care for a disabled spouse. In her study of a group of informal carers, Ungerson (1987) suggests that the men she interviewed used the language of love, none of them making any reference to 'duty':

'I love her – it's as simple as that! I promised at my wedding; I meant the vows at the time and will always mean them.' (Mr Vaughan, caring for his disabled wife, in Ungerson, 1987)

However, of the women Ungerson (1987) spoke to, although some referred to the love they had for their husbands, all alluded to their sense of duty.

This highlights the gender differences in the formation of caring relationships, for it would appear that men are most likely to care *for* those they care *about*. Women, however, will be led by normative socialization towards the obligation of caring *for* those who they feel have legitimate claim on their sense of duty, which can be generalized, and shift from one relationship to another (Ungerson, 1987: 92).

PARENTS AS CAREGIVERS

On the whole, parents are expected by society to assume responsibility for the survival and healthy development of their children. It is mainly mothers who are the most significantly involved in this nurturing role. However, parents often experience the anxiety brought about by parenthood. This is expressed by a new father, after his new baby daughter had to be resuscitated following a traumatic delivery:

And I thought, 'Oh gosh, is this what having a kid is like? Terrors like this? Will she be okay tomorrow? Will she be okay the day after?'
(Bergum, 1989: 31)

For those parents whose children are not 'okay', born with, or going on to develop a physical illness, handicap or learning disability, the 'normal' parental anxiety can become long-term and last a lifetime.

After the birth of a baby, parents, particularly mothers, of children who have a disability will often be the first to suspect that 'something is wrong'. When medical professionals confirm suspicions, parents will usually have to confront feelings of grief, associated with the loss of the 'normal' child they did not have. Because of the stigma surrounding disability, their grief will be compounded by guilt, a sense of failure and loss of self-esteem (Hicks, 1988).

Research has indicated that most of the care of children with disabilities is undertaken by mothers, with little help from other members of the family (Parker, 1990). When considering 'care in the community', a study by Wilkin (1979) also indicated that a very heavy burden is carried by mothers, with very little support given by networks of friends and neighbours, or in other words 'the community'. More recently, the nature of parents' caregiving has changed. Parents of chronically sick children at home frequently perform complex and highly technical nursing procedures with variable support from community nurses (Kirk and Glendinning, 1998).

Mothers can demonstrate a high level of commitment and feel a powerful bond to sick and disabled children. Pat, who has a supportive family and cares for her daughter of 12 who is severely handicapped with a mental age of five months, says:

I centre my life around Vicky. I don't know what I'll do when she dies ... the joy has outweighed the anguish and she has been such a pleasure and delight to all of us who know and love her.

(Briggs and Oliver, 1985: 15)

On the whole, the parents of children with a disability are no different from the parents of 'normal' children in wanting to help them develop their potential as far as possible, and to prepare them for an independent life. This desire to foster independence despite disability could be said to reflect the world view of individualistic, medicalized, Western society, seeking normalization at all cost.

When considering parents from different cultures as informal carers, Anderson and Elfert (1989) focused on the experiences of immigrant Chinese as well as white middle-class families who cared for chronically ill children in Canada. These authors' findings highlight the different perceptions of caring between the two groups. Chinese parents' expression of caring for their disabled children was to foster happiness and contentment, not to inflict discomfort and distress by rigorous stimulation and exercise. On the other hand, Anglo-Canadian parents readily embraced the ideology of normalization, which permeates Canadian and other Western cultures. They point out that these immigrant Chinese families, particularly the non-English-speaking women, were often socially isolated from the mainstream society and the ideological structure of the Canadian health care system. It is possible that a similar difference could be identified among some new immigrant groups in the UK.

There are children with disabilities from every culture, who will grow up to become independent of their parents. However, some will continue to need care from their families as long as they live. This can mean that some parents will remain in their caring role well into their old age, living with the anxiety and uncertainty of their adult child's future, once they are unable to care.

It has been estimated that there are 10 000 elderly parents caring for middle-aged disabled offspring, some of whom have spent much of their adult life as carers (Hicks, 1988). Others, however, will have taken on the care of their adult offspring following the onset of a chronic illness or an accident.

At the age of 25, Richard Hughes, now 52, contracted diabetes, and returned to his parents with whom he has lived for the past 27 years. His illness has proved to be very unstable, and as a result he has not been able to work and has had to have a leg amputated. His parents, now in their 80s are tired, themselves both suffering from chronic illnesses, yet they still feel responsible for his welfare. They are both experts on the management of diabetes and continue to monitor the balance between glucose and insulin that keeps their son alive. When referring to Richard's frequent 'hypo's' his father, Owen Hughes, says:

> I'm getting too old, and the wife's getting too old to cope with it, you see. He doesn't know he's doing it. He'll call you all the names out, and he's so strong, he can hit me over! I've got some special stuff, although I'm a bit clumsy, which I can inject into his arm. But he's got to be unconscious. With his arms flying, you can't do it, you see. You try to undress him, to inject him, but very often I can't do it now . . . (cited in McClure, 1993: 20)

The long-term caregiving of parents of adult children with a disability can result in dependent or conflict-ridden relationships and, in her research, Walmsley (1996, cited in Brechin *et al.*, 1998) argues for service provision which does not bind families into long-term interdependence for 'better or worse' (p. 399). However, family caregivers can be excluded from discussions about the future of the cared-for, leading to disagreements between professionals and parents (Brechin *et al.*, 1998).

OFFSPRING AS CAREGIVERS

It has been suggested that within modern British society it is normal for adult children to feel responsible for the care of their parents should it become necessary. This reflects one view that family relationships have a special moral character which is expressed as 'caring without reckoning' or, in other words, without counting the cost (Bloch, 1973). However, as is evident in the case of those caring for other close kin, the care of an aged and disabled lone parent is mostly undertaken by daughters; sons, on the whole, being exempted by society due to their usual role as the main breadwinner. The caring role of sons will often be demonstrated by their financing of parental care (Dalley, 1988). When finances are not available, or formal care inappropriate, it is suggested that families will tend to negotiate caring responsibilities between their members, taking into account their circumstances and life-course stages (Finch, 1987). Yet the full burden of day-to-day care of lone elderly and infirm parents tends to fall upon a single family member, usually a daughter or daughter-in-law, regardless of her employment status (Albert, 1990).

There are more married women caring for parents due to the rise in marriage rates over the last 30 years, but there are still about 300 000 single women living with elderly parents, of whom 156 000 have a major caring role. Although not torn between social roles and responsibilities like her married counterpart, the single daughter has, in the past been likely to lose both financial and social independence.

Married daughters have different problems. They can find their loyalties divided between the demands of their husbands and children, and the parent or parent-in-law they care for, which can take its toll on both their physical and mental health:

> I couldn't see my mum in a home – it would break my heart. My husband I love equally. Who is more important in the end? (Julie Beale, 53, caring for her mother since she was 13, through 30 years of married life, in Hicks, 1988: 40)

Caring for an elderly parent within a home designed for the nuclear family can lead to conflict between the generations, with the 'woman of the house' having to try to keep the peace. Husbands vary in the amount of help they will offer, even if the receiver of care is their parent. Privacy between husband and wife can be disrupted, and wives can be torn between the demands of the elderly parent and those of children, who at this stage are often facing the problems of adolescence. The deterioration of an elderly parent's physical or mental condition, resulting in incontinence or dementia, can lead to acute anxiety within a three-generation family, for, in this society, it is commonly believed that children should not be exposed to the painful realities of ageing and death (Hicks, 1988).

Married daughters from ethnic minorities have the same problems as their indigenous counterparts. These can be compounded by isolation in a foreign country, language difficulties and lack of experience of how to seek help from agencies often ill-equipped to meet their needs. The problems of Black elderly people from ethnic minorities were highlighted in a report funded by the Department of Health and Social Security (DHSS) (Norman, 1985). However, their carers remain 'one of the most neglected and invisible groups in the country' and there is as yet little research into the experiences of Asian and Afro-Caribbean caregivers (Ahmed and Atkin, 1996).

But it is not always adult offspring who find themselves in the caring role. Research by Aldridge and Becker (1993) and Dearden and Becker (1998) indicates that there are school-age children who are known to have the responsibility of caring for a disabled parent. The research by Aldridge and Becker (1993), undertaken in Nottingham, raised public awareness of the experience of young carers under the age of 16. More recent research has estimated that, nationally, between 19 000 and 51 000 children are caregivers (Walker, 1996). All studies related to young caregivers indicate that many were socialized into their caring role from a very early age, and that their caring role could affect their health and development (Frank et al., 1999).

Debra, aged 16, has cared for her mother who has Huntington's chorea since the age of 12, and says:

> I didn't feel as I'd had any choice, but it didn't bother me – I'd been used to it since I was so young. Sometimes it gets to you – not very often 'cos I'm used to it.
>
> (Aldridge and Becker, 1993)

Within this research, most of the young caregivers were girls, which reinforces previous research about gender and caring. Four out of six of the boys were of Asian origin, which might demonstrate the cultural expectations that caring remains within the family, outside intervention not being sought. However, it is also possible that statutory agencies were inaccessible to these families.

The nature of caring undertaken by all 15 of these children ranged from domestic chores, such as cleaning, cooking and shopping to personal care, which included lifting, bathing and toileting. It is evident that tasks such as lifting were often too much for the young caregiver, especially as none of them had any instruction in lifting techniques. Claire, aged 15, who has cared for her immobile mother since she was 12, carries her 'piggy back' up two flights of stairs to the bedroom and bathroom. She describes how:

> I fell with my Mum like because I've got a bad knee. I bruised a tendon and had a lot of shit done on my knee and that, so I'm not supposed to carry her, but I still do it.
>
> (Aldridge and Becker, 1993: 26)

Young caregivers will perform intimate caring tasks because there appears to be no alternative, but they express distaste for their involvement. Miriam, now age 29, has cared from the age of 15 for her mother who has multiple sclerosis:

> I used to hate seeing her naked. I hadn't seen an older woman like that. I know it's my mother but it's just something you don't do, you don't see your mother naked.
>
> (Aldridge and Becker, 1993: 27)

Implicit in all the experiences related above, family caregivers of both sexes, of all ages, and from every culture are usually engaged in private, domestic and often invisible work, dutifully fulfilling both their own and their society's expectations of their various roles within family and community.

Research has, in the past, focused on the difficulties experienced by carers implying the burden of caring (Atkin and Rollings, 1996) but there is growing evidence that caregiving within a loving relationship can also offer satisfactions that may contribute towards individual coping mechanisms (Nolan *et al.*, 1996).

Nurses working with their clients in the community will have direct and indirect contact with caregivers of every type, within homes and clinics, surgeries and schools. Official rhetoric implies that community nurses and family caregivers can work in partnership, together providing the formal and informal caring required by those cared for. In an attempt to ground rhetoric in reality, this proposed partnership will now be explored within a framework suggested by Twigg (1989), and adapted to include the concept of the 'expert' caregiver.

Community nurses' relationships with carers

'Partnership' is a buzzword, used liberally in contemporary health care literature. A partnership suggests a particular relationship, encompassing mutual recognition and respect and a degree of equality in status. Twigg (1989), examined how social care agencies conceptualize their relationships with informal carers and identified three models:

- A resource.
- Co-workers.
- Co-clients.

Following many years of research into the experiences of informal carers, Nolan *et al.* (1996) suggest a fourth model of carers as experts, which could result in a perception by community nurses as co-experts. This section will consider the relationships that community nurses can have with family caregivers within each of these models, in an attempt to explore to what extent a partnership between them is possible.

FAMILY CAREGIVERS AS A RESOURCE – PARTNERSHIP OR EXPLOITATION?

It has been demonstrated by the experiences of the caregivers referred to earlier, that they are, indeed, a resource according to the estimation that their services save the taxpayer £33 billion each year (Nuttall, 1992). But, community nurses can regard family caregivers as 'the given', being taken for granted, as a resource around which the service is structured. This is illustrated by Briggs and Oliver (1985) in their account of the experiences of 20 carers:

> The nurse expects the family carer to be in the house when she arrives, and frequently requires the help of the carer for tasks like lifting, which nurses are not allowed to undertake by themselves, though the carer is seldom aided in this!'
>
> (Briggs and Oliver, 1985: 110)

This hardly suggests a partnership, for the carer's contribution is not always acknowledged or recognized. Within this model, family caregivers of all ages, who are able to cope without complaint, tend to be ignored, intervention being offered only when there is a crisis (Kirk and Glendinning, 1998). Their morale is not considered (Richardson, 1998) and conflicts of interest between the caregiver and the cared-for can often be overlooked (Twigg, 1989). Despite recent legislation (DOH, 1996, 1999b), they are still not consistently acknowledged as legitimate recipients of the community nursing service (Henwood, 1998) and their role is frequently overlooked altogether (CNA, 1998).

But it could be that carers do not always see *themselves* as legitimate recipients of community nursing care. British society is medicalized, placing a high value on the curative capacity of medical science. Historically, Western societies have systematically presented health care practice in a way that gives high rewards and superior status to the doctor who cures, the low status caring component of healing being undervalued or disregarded (Versluysen, 1980). Although known as the 'caring profession', many aspects of nursing are associated by the public with biomedicine, which is focused on the treatment of those with conditions diagnosed by doctors.

Nurses and family caregivers alike will acknowledge that caregiving is not a disease with a medical diagnosis, associated with a prescribed treatment. Therefore it is possible that neither nurse nor carer is likely to consider caring as an activity which warrants professional nursing assessment and intervention. Within this model carers, too, could see themselves as a resource, their duty and obligation reinforced by cultural and moral influences, as well as by social policy committed to reducing public expenditure (Bridges and Lynam, 1993). Only time will tell if the Carers Services and Recognition Act (1996) and the national strategy for carers (DOH, 1999a) can change these public perceptions and elevate the status of caring to equal that of curative medicine.

FAMILY CAREGIVERS AND COMMUNITY NURSES AS CO-WORKERS – CAN THIS BE CALLED A PARTNERSHIP?

This perspective implies a partnership between family caregivers and community nurses, both working together to provide care for family members and clients. Twigg (1989) suggests that within this model, the role of carers is acknowledged, but their health and well-being are only considered within the context of being able to continue caring. There is evidence that many who cope successfully with their caring role work closely with nurses, often taking on what can be considered to be nursing duties:

I help the nurse when she comes. I'm what they call the dirty nurse. I tear all the packets, its all got to be sterile . . . three years more or less, I've dressed it myself at night. I don't irrigate the wound, but I clean it and all that . . . (Mrs Darby, who cares for her disabled husband, in Parker, 1993:18)

It seems that Mrs Darby is seen, not so much as a co-worker but as the junior, the dirty nurse who helps the qualified nurse, but who lacks the training and confidence to undertake a sterile dressing. Parker (1990) also refers to the discriminatory nature of some community nursing service provision. Arber *et al.* (1988) found that 'elderly who are co-resident with younger married women are least likely to receive district nursing service'.

When considering carers from ethnic minorities, there can be the assumption that coming from societies, which have a less individualistic and more communal way of life, 'they look after their own'. What can be overlooked, though, is that many of these ethnic caregivers (usually women) do not always have access to the social networks available to them in their homeland (Hicks, 1988). Many of those who are second- or third-generation will have jobs outside the home and the same aspirations as their indigenous peers. Recent immigrants, who are ignorant of, and ignored by a service insensitive to their needs, are unlikely to benefit from the help available to them. This suggests that the opportunity of access to a community nurse as a co-worker can also be unequal, dependent on the gender, age and ethnic background of the carer.

What community nurses and family caregivers share as co-workers in caring, is the emotional and physical stresses both encounter in their daily work (Hicks, 1988; Smith, 1992). However, at this level, as co-workers or partners, professional nurses could be said to have the clear advantage. The vast majority will have chosen their occupation and will have access to the acquisition of the knowledge, skills and attitudes whereby they can fulfil their role. They will have opportunity for further education, career advancement, and paid holidays and pension rights. Unlike the majority of family caregivers, they thus have security, recognized status and a degree of power within society, and can choose the extent of their personal involvement. The status of qualified nurses may remain lower than that of doctors, society considering the value of professional caring lower than that of curing. But the value placed on family caregiving is lower still.

If nursing has been likened to the individualized arm of the public health movement (Dunlop, 1986) then family caregiving can be likened to unseen tireless hands behind the scenes, which are only noticed once they are no longer able to function. Community nurses and carers do work together as co-workers, but the inequalities demonstrated above, indicate that their collaboration cannot be considered to be a true and equal partnership.

FAMILY CAREGIVERS AS CO-CLIENTS OF COMMUNITY NURSES – PARTNERSHIP PREVENTING CRISIS?

Within this model, carers would no longer be seen by community nurses as a resource to be exploited, or co-workers to be co-opted. They become the responsibility of the community nursing service, their needs being assessed separately from those of their dependants. This could lead to recognition of the possible conflicts of interest between caregivers' needs and those of the cared-for. This can result in either the subsequent termination of their caring activity or continuous nursing support should they choose to carry on.

When asked about community nursing initiatives in the support of family caregivers, a community mental health nurse clearly sees them as co-clients:

> We aim to identify and help to meet their needs, as we believe family caregivers are equally important as our patients. We will often visit them alone to help, support and to offer advice to enable them to continue caring or to support them in decision making for future care.

This view is supported by the comment of a community nurse working with people with learning difficulties, who says:

> . . . in the field the caregiver is the client, in as much as it is his/her needs which are being addressed in relation to caring for their relative at home.

These nurses appear to have developed a concept of partnership with carers within this model. Their comments suggest mutual understanding and an open consideration of their needs reflecting obligation and responsibility.

However, Neale (1993), when referring to the needs of those caring for someone with a terminal illness, suggests that there is little evidence in practice that this model is consistently adopted early enough to prevent carer exhaustion or burnout. In a more recent study, Brown and Stetz (1999) found that formal health care providers rarely acknowledge the contributions that are made in the care of those terminally ill.

As well as the differences expressed above, Twigg (1989) suggests that perceptions of carer as co-client can impinge upon the normal processes of life, on the one hand; swamping the services with 'human misery', on the other. In some cases, its use appears to be confined to those who reach a physical or psychological breaking point. This could mean that the caregiver may well become a client, and within the medical understanding of stress a legitimate recipient of nursing intervention. This will imply the kind of partnership reserved for clients, the nature of which, it can be argued, can also be based upon an unequal relationship.

It is therefore illustrated from the above three models, that community nurses' perceptions of and relationships with family caregivers can be fraught with practical ambiguities and not always the straightforward partnership so readily assumed and confidently exhorted in recent literature and legislation. In their research, Nolan et al. (1996) acknowledge that these models can in some cases be appropriate. But they propose that it is the primary model 'co-experts' that can most aptly be applied to community nurses and caregivers and which implies a more explicit and equal partnership.

FAMILY CAREGIVERS AND COMMUNITY NURSES AS CO-EXPERTS: LEARNING TOGETHER?

Benner (1984) highlighted the concept of 'expertise' and defines the expert as someone who 'operates from a deep understanding of the total situation' (p. 32) and who 'rapidly grasps the problem by seeing it in relation to past similar and dissimilar situations and rapidly hones in on the correct region of the problem' (p. 215). This definition from the nursing literature could lead to the assumption that, as professionals, all experienced nurses achieve 'expert' status. Similarly, there could be the assumption that as members of the lay public, family caregivers will need to be facilitated by these expert nurses in order to achieve co-expert status. However, by considering this definition in context, it could equally apply to some experienced family caregivers as well as to some experienced community nurses or, on the other hand, depending on the context, to neither.

Family caregivers as experts

In their research into the experiences of the caregivers during a potentially fatal illness, Brown and Stetz (1999) found that the initial willingness to care:

> Often depended on several factors, including the sense of obligation and reciprocity, the degree of conflict or intimacy in the relationship and what the care recipient would allow to occur, and what the caregiver was willing to give.
>
> (Brown and Stetz, 1999: 188)

This implies that even at the start of a caregiving relationship, the caregiver has an in-depth understanding of the particular situation, based on knowledge about the individual cared for, and his or her biographical history. But this can depend on a range of variables such as age, relationship, the nature of disability and the availability of information about the disease or disability.

It could be argued that there is a significant level of expertise amongst experienced family caregivers (Kirk and Glendinning, 1998). It has been found that they have a 'very strong sense of their own expertise' (Nolan et al., 1999: 196), but this is often acquired over time, through a process of trial and error (Brown and Stetz, 1999; Nolan et al., 1999) and often without significant support from community nurses.

COMMUNITY NURSES AS EXPERTS

Since 1998 (or earlier for some), nurses who have undertaken a post-registration qualification in one of the eight specialisms in community nursing will qualify from their degree-level courses as competent specialist practitioners (UKCC, 1994). As registered professionals with an additional qualification, community nurses will be equipped with a comprehensive overview, their professional knowledge being a synthesis of evidence-based theory and professional experience. Although answerable to the UK Central Council for nursing, midwifery and health visiting via the professional code of conduct (UKCC, 1992), it can be argued that expert community nursing practice, like expert family caregiving is also likely to depend on a range of variables. Prior experience, length of experience, professional priorities, level of autonomy and available resources are but a few of the issues that can influence community nursing expertise in working with family caregivers.

The learning needs of family caregivers and community nurses in acquiring expertise

A framework proposed by Nolan and Grant (1989), looks at some of the self-identified needs of family caregivers which tend not to be met by professionals. By adapting this framework, the concept of 'support' is broken down into three specific areas which can be related to caregivers and community nurses alike, and which might, if addressed, enhance the expertise of both. These can be defined as:

- Information.
- Skills.
- Emotional support.

INFORMATION NEEDS OF FAMILY CAREGIVERS

When chronic sickness or disability is diagnosed, individuals and families can enter into foreign territory, finding themselves in unfamiliar places inhabited by strange people who speak a partially understood language. Words such as *cancer, cerebral vascular accident, multiple sclerosis, incontinence, schizophrenia, cerebral palsy* and *Down's syndrome* can fill them with dread and uncertainty. A diagnosis might have been confirmed at a hospital, surgery or clinic where pressure of time or the initial shock could have inhibited the absorption of information given, as well as the formulation of pertinent questions. It is once they return home, that fears can be articulated into questions which are likely to include: 'How will this condition progress?' 'How will we cope?' 'Who can help?' These are questions which require discussion and, where possible, answers if immediate needs are to be met and long-term plans considered by users and carers alike. It can be argued that community nurses can often be the most appropriate of health and social care professionals to provide the information required. They are familiar with the territory and speak the medical language.

John Peters needed more information following the discovery that his new baby had Down's syndrome:

... and I didn't even know what Down's syndrome was then, 'What's that?' I said, and the doctor didn't put it very well. He told us, 'Your little boy will never be normal' ... and I walked away from the hospital and my mind was a blank.

(McClure, 1993: 32)

When a parent is a carer, it is reasonable to expect that community nurses who work with children, will be able to give parents information about the child's condition. Yet a survey undertaken by Meltzer, Smythe and Robus (1989, cited in Parker, 1990), found that levels of health visiting to parents of disabled children were lower than expected, and that community nursing involvement with these children and their parents, was significantly less than that with adults. It was found that the parents of the most severely disabled children considered this shortfall in community nursing service to be one of their most significant unmet needs.

Ethical dilemmas concerning issues of confidentiality may arise when a family carer asks community nurses working with adults about diagnosis and prognosis. This will require a high level of diplomacy, if the community nurse is simultaneously to meet the needs of both caregiver and cared-for. However, in most instances caregivers need accurate information in order to fully appreciate the situation (Brown and Stetz, 1999). This could serve to reduce hostility between caregiver and cared-for (Nolan and Grant, 1989) and to facilitate informed choice about the possibility and extent of their future involvement. Modern technology has ensured that the lay public has access to much medical information – and to much misinformation. Community nurses are in a position to give accurate, evidence-based and up-to-date medical information to carers, but information-giving or, in other words, teaching and advocacy takes time and specialized skills. A carer with questions might not see fit to ask a community nurse who appears busy and distracted (Ong, 1990) and if the information needs of carers are not a community nurse's priority, questions might not be invited.

It is also of importance to carers that they have access to information about relevant services for they are often unaware of where to get hold of the information they need (Brown and Stetz, 1999). In a survey undertaken by the Carer's National Association (CNA) in 1998, one carer asked:

Why do carers have to find out any information about help by asking around people in similar circumstances as themselves, and not getting the information from people like benefit offices, clinics and hospitals?

(CNA, 1998: 5)

INFORMATION NEEDS OF COMMUNITY NURSES

Community nurses are expected to know how to deliver effective care to meet the health needs of individual patients. As an advocate of family nursing which is just starting to be acknowledged in British nursing, Whyte (1997) suggests that nurses could lack the theoretical knowledge required in order to provide family nursing interventions at three levels. These are to individuals within a family context, at the interpersonal level within family relationships and at the level of the whole family system. It could be argued, too, that within each specific situation, families themselves, who could have a deep understanding of the total situation, would, if consulted, be able to provide the accurate and relevant information required for effective community nursing interventions.

Community nurses will need the confidence to seek information from both caregivers and patients about how the illness or disability they live with affects their lives. They will also need to be able to access information about the wide range of acute and chronic illnesses and disabilities, and in knowing their patients or caregivers, be able to both answer and ask questions appropriately. This will mean keeping up to date with constantly changing medical and nursing knowledge and evidence-based practice. Similarly, all nurses working in the community are required to compile community profiles (Tinson, 1995). Through this process of community needs assessment, they will gain a comprehensive knowledge of the national and local statutory and voluntary agencies that target the needs of those with chronic illness and disabilities, and their caregivers.

SKILLS NEEDS OF FAMILY CAREGIVERS

As illustrated throughout this chapter, informal carers of all ages can be involved with a wide range of personal care, involving the skills usually undertaken by trained nurses. These can include washing, bathing, lifting, incontinence care and the administration of medication. More invasive procedures can also be carried out, such as the giving of injections, urinary catheterization, bladder washouts and manual bowel evacuations. Qualified community nurses, as experienced practitioners and teachers, are well-equipped to impart all these skills to appropriate carers. However, Atkinson (1992), in his paper which studied the nursing support which informal carers provided for disabled dependants, found that very few of the carers he interviewed had received any instruction in the nursing procedures they undertook. He describes how carers can drift into situations which could be considered to be unacceptable to professional health care workers because of the health risks involved to both carers and cared-for. Situations such as these have been referred to earlier in the accounts of the young carers injured through lifting their parents. Another is cited in Atkinson (1992) where the 15-year-old son of a woman severely disabled with multiple sclerosis carried out regular manual bowel evacuations for his mother. It is likely that community nurses would avoid teaching these young carers the correct way in which to perform these procedures because of the risk of physical and emotional damage. But given a situation where no other help is available, a lack of instruction will also carry risks.

The same could apply to older carers in poor health required to undertake heavy lifting. It can be seen therefore that the skills' training which carers require is not always straightforward and can present community nurses with complex dilemmas. The limited number of qualified community nurses available to focus on the effective teaching of carers can compound this complexity. The fact that some carers are taking on an inappropriate nursing role in the first place could reflect this deficit in the service.

SKILLS NEEDS OF COMMUNITY NURSES

These dilemmas are likely to become more commonplace as more children and adults with chronic illness and disabilities are cared for in the community. Community nurses working as co-experts with family caregivers will be alert to their needs and will need to enhance their assessment skills to include complex family dynamics. They will need to be familiar with theories of adult education and be skilled in identifying learning needs and in facilitating appropriate learning. To achieve this as specialist practitioners they will need to be able to engage in complex and autonomous decision-making and become informed advocates. They will need to work closely with leaders who provide health care in the community, indicating possibilities and creative solutions, as well as shortfalls and dangers within the service. But this, too, requires a commitment to carers' needs, the necessary education and the willingness to 'secularize' professional nursing skills, where appropriate, and to facilitate the developing expertise of family caregivers without withdrawing altogether once this is achieved.

EMOTIONAL NEEDS OF FAMILY CAREGIVERS

The nature of care undertaken by family caregivers will vary considerably from the rewarding and satisfying to the physically taxing and emotionally draining. All carers, because of the often-unremitting nature of their work, are likely either constantly, or from time to time, to suffer varying degrees of frustration and emotional distress.

Those caregivers who gain expertise through the acquisition of relevant information and skill are likely to feel more valued, recognized and in control of their situation, which could raise their self-esteem. However, in the long term, the self-esteem and endurance of the most committed carer can become eroded. Feeling trapped, unable to carry on, and unable to hand over to anyone else, some can be driven to breaking point, which can lead to a physical or psychological breakdown or to violence directed at their dependant.

Pat Watman, when caring for her elderly mother who suffers from dementia, describes her feelings:

Few people can understand the sense of desperation, left alone for long periods with a confused elderly person, unless they have done it themselves. It makes you do and say cruel things even though you love the person. That's when it is dangerous. I loved her, but she unwittingly drove me over the brink – into violence. At first it was just verbal, but then I started to hit her, and pull her around, and throw her on the bed . . .

(Hicks, 1988: 65)

In a survey by Ogg *et al.* (1991 in Laurent, 1993), of 2130 carers and dependants interviewed, 10% of carers admitted abuse and 5% of the elderly people being cared for reported being abused.

Individuals can begin their caring out of love or duty to partner, offspring or parent, but over time, they can find themselves subjugated to the caring role. Locked into a caring relationship that can marginalize their own needs, they see no alternatives. Throughout their caring career it is likely that both themselves and others have directed the focus of attention unremittingly on the needs of the cared-for. It is hardly surprising that they then fail to recognize their own physical and mental health needs. The daily grind of unrelieved caring for someone they love can swing between resentment and guilt, leading to various forms of depression and hopelessness. This could make it difficult to 'let go' and relinquish the burden of care. Therefore even if it were available, some carers might find it difficult to accept relief and respite.

Social isolation is commonly felt by informal carers of all ages. Because of the demands that caregiving makes on their time, and the anxieties they have about leaving their dependants unattended, caregivers can become alienated from and lose touch with their non-caring peers who are unable to understand their situation.

A way in which community nurses can intervene in order to raise the self-esteem of carers, and to reduce their feelings of isolation, is by the facilitation of carer self-help groups. These groups are often initiated by community workers, social workers and voluntary organizations, but there is some evidence that they are also being run by community nurses 'working in a different way', as suggested by Bridges and Lynam (1993). In a small opportunistic survey of 97 community nurses from five specialities, working within nine different fund holding trusts and surgeries 40% were aware of community nurse involvement in carers' support groups. It can be assumed that meeting with others can help to alleviate the isolation, giving carers an opportunity to talk and listen to those in the same position.

One exploratory study by Morton and Mackenzie (1994) suggests that members do find the group a valuable source of mutual and social support. The Carers National Association (CNA) has recently published a primary care projects directory, in which 68 carers' projects across the country are listed, offering information, support and advice (CNA, 1998). Projects offering support for young caregivers have developed nationwide since 1995, 123 of these having been listed in 1997. Abigail (age 15) sums up the nature of the support these can provide:

It's given me the chance to know who's in the same position as me, and for me to talk to someone that I know can relate to me, because they've either been through it, of they are going through it.

(Dearden and Becker, 1998: 54)

But self-support groups are not appropriate for all carers. Some will find it difficult to attend, as they are unable to leave their dependant for any length of time. Others have no wish to spend precious time listening to other people's problems and men might feel out of place in a predominantly female group.

Community nurses are likely to be in contact with carers when assessing the needs of their clients and during the implementation of their nursing assessment. They will also be aware of the recovery or death of their clients. During these contacts, it would appear expedient, in the light of carers' expressed needs, to invite carers to talk about their own emotional needs. But this would take time, extend the length of each visit and, it may be argued, overburden a finite service. Community nurses themselves, as autonomous practitioners, would need to acknowledge this intervention as a priority health need. And if community nurses are to provide significant emotional support to family caregivers, how are they prepared and what kind of emotional support is available to them?

EMOTIONAL SKILLS AND NEEDS OF COMMUNITY NURSES

If family caregivers become overstretched or 'burnt out', community nurses working alongside as co-experts will need to draw on advanced assessment and listening skills as well as intuitive judgement based on their knowledge of the situation. They would be well-placed to advocate respite to enable the caregiver to continue caring subsequently (Weightman, 1999). The ability to facilitate carers' groups, or to work with others to do so, could be a creative response to the needs of carers within a community. But to be effectively engaged in this, community nurses are themselves likely to need their own support, which in the light of recent developments in nursing might be available in the form of regular clinical supervision.

Smith (1992) called for further research into the area of emotion and health care. More recently, clinical supervision, having had its origins in psychiatry, counselling and social work, is slowly being developed within nursing (Butterworth et al., 1998). It is suggested that clinical supervision should enable nurses to reflect on issues which affect practice, to learn from experience, to problem-solve and to identify ways of dealing with difficult emotions. An explanation for the cautious response that nurses have had to clinical supervision could lie in the term itself. This could carry meanings which reflect a management agenda associated with control and authority. Nurses might also have fears about acknowledging their emotions, and developing their own potential for power and autonomy (Bond and Holland, 1998). The urgent need for clinical supervision aptly noted by Swain (1995) is highly relevant when considering the needs of community nurses working as co-experts with family caregivers:

It beggars belief that we have for so long, failed to incorporate (clinical supervision) as a defined component of practice. Any one of us looking back at the human pain and social distress of others to which we have been exposed – not to mention our own – must surely question what makes us suppose we can practice effectively without such a regular conscious examination of our work, of what might improve it, what might impede it and of our own feelings about it.

(Swain, 1995: 12)

Conclusion

Continuing advances in medical science and technology are likely to enable more chronically sick and disabled people of all ages to live in their own homes. Some disabled people will have the opportunity to take charge of their own care and become 'expert patients'. Where necessary, they will be able to arrange and purchase their own personal assistance through the Direct Payments Bill (1996). But there will be others who at various times will require husbands, wives, lovers, children, parents and friends to provide care, ranging from mundane domestic help to highly technical and invasive nursing procedures. It follows that caregivers will be required also to become expert in what they do for the safety, comfort and well being of cared-for and caregivers alike.

The medical model of health care has saved countless people of all ages for a life of chronic disability, and there is evidence that they, if given the chance, can live fulfilled lives. Government legislation has responded to the needs of disabled people (DSS, 1996; DoH, 1999) some of whom are now able to become experts in their own care. The needs of caregivers are now recognized at government level, and they are officially entitled to support (DOH, 1996, 1999).

Recent legislation (DOH, 1997, 1999a) indicates that nurses could now be in a position to start moving away from the restrictions of this same medical model, to take it further and promote their long-held vision of holistic nursing care. As representatives in PCGs or PCTs and as nurse consultants, they are well-placed to have an influence in promoting the value of continuing care of patients and clients within a family and community setting.

For, if community nurses are going to be able to work with family caregivers as co-experts, it will be necessary to learn to focus on families, to become skilled facilitators of learning and to be prepared to recognize their own supervision needs when providing emotional support.

Above all, as lifelong learners their practice will be enhanced if they can acknowledge and learn from that caring ethos borrowed by their own profession, which has been, and always will be securely rooted in the enduring care that takes place within family relationships.

References

Ahmed, W.I.U. and Adkin, K. (1996) *'Race' and community care*. Buckingham: Open University Press.

Albert, S.M. (1990) Care giving as a cultural system in urban America. *American Ethnologist*, 192: 319–31.

Aldridge, J. and Becker, S. (1993) *Children who care*. Leicestershire: Loughborough University Department of Social Science.

Anderson, J. and Elfert, H. (1989) Managing chronic illness in the family: women as caretakers. *Journal of Advanced Nursing*, 14: 735–43.

Arber, S., Gilbert, N. and Evandrou, M. (1988) Gender household composition, and receipt of domiciliary services by the elderly disabled. *Journal of Social Policy*, 17: 153–75.

Arber, S. and Ginn, J. (1990a) The meaning of informal care: gender and the contribution of elderly people. *Ageing and Society*, 10: 429–54.

Arber, S. and Ginn, J. (1990b) In sickness and in health: care-giving, gender and the independence of elderly people. In: Marsh, C. and Arber, S. (eds) *Households and families: divisions and change*. London: Macmillan.

Atkinson, F.I. (1992) Experiences of informal carers providing nursing support for disabled dependants. *Journal of Advanced Nursing*, 17: 835–40.

Atkin, K. and Rollings, J. (1996) Looking after their own. In: Ahmed, W.I.U. and Atkin, K. *Race and community care*. Milton Keynes: Open University Press.

Benner, P. (1984) *From novice to expert: excellence and power in clinical nursing*. California: Addison-Wesley.

Bergum, V. (1989) *Woman to mother*. Massachusetts: Bergin & Garvey Inc.

Bloch, M. (1973) The long term and the short term: the economics and political significance of the morality of kinship. In: Goody, J. (ed.) *The character of kinship*. Cambridge: Cambridge University Press.

Bond, M. and Holland, S. (1997) *Skills of clinical supervision for nurses: a practical guide for clinical supervisors and managers*. Buckingham: Open University Press.

Brechin, A., Walmsley, J., Katz, J. and Peace, S. (eds.) (1998) *Care matters*. London: Sage.

Bridges, J. and Lynam, M. (1993) Informal carers: a Marxist analysis of social, political and economic forces underpinning the role. *Advanced Nursing Science*, 15: 33–48.

Briggs, A. and Oliver, J. (1985) *Caring, experiences of looking after disabled relatives*. London: Routledge & Kegan Paul.

Brown, M. and Stetz, K. (1999) The labour of caregiving: a theoretical model of caregiving during potentially fatal illness. *Qualitative Health Research*, 9: 182–97.

Butterworth, T., Faughier, J. and Burnard, P. (eds) *Clinical supervision and mentorship in nursing*. Cheltenham: Stanley Thomas.

Carers National Aassociation. (1998) *The new carers' code*. London: CNA.

Department of Health and Social Security. (1981) Growing older. In: Parker, G. *With due care and attention, a review of research on informal care*. London: Family Policy Studies Centre.

Dalley, G. (1988) *Ideologies of caring*. London: Macmillan.

Dearden, C. and Becker, S. (1998) *Young carers in the UK*. Loughborough University: Young Carers Research Group.

Department of Health. (1989) *Caring for people. Community care in the next decade and beyond*. London: HMSO.

Department of Health. (1990) *The NHS and community care act*. London: HMSO.

Department of Heatlh. (1996) *The carers (recognition and services) act.* London: HMSO.

Department of Health. (1997) *The new NHS – modern and dependable.* London: The Stationery Office.

Department of Health. (1999a) *Caring for carers. A national strategy for carers.* London: The Stationery Office.

Department of Health. (1999b) *Saving lives – our healthier nation.* London: The Stationery Office.

Dunlop, M. (1986) Is a science of caring possible? Journal of Advanced Nursing, 11: 661–70.

Family Policy Bulletin (1989) In: *An income policy for carers.* (1992). London: Caring Costs.

Finch, J. (1987) Family obligations and the life course. In: Bryman, A. et al. (eds) *Rethinking the life cycle.* Basingstoke: Macmillan.

Frank, J., Tatum, C. and Tucker, S. (1999) *On small shoulders: learning from the experiences of former young carers.* London: The Children's Society.

Henwood, M. (1998) *Ignored and invisible?* London: CNA.

Hicks, C. (1988) *Who cares: looking after people at home.* London: Virago.

Kirk, S. and Glendinning, C. (1998) Trends in community care and patient participation: implications for the roles of informal carers and community nurses in the United Kingdom. *Journal of Advanced Nursing,* 28: 370–81.

Laurent, C. (1993) Age old problem. *Nursing Times,* 89: 9 June.

Lawler, J. (1991) *Behind the screens: nursing, somology and the problem of the body.* London: Churchill Livingstone.

Lister, P. (1997) The art of nursing in a 'post modern' context. *Journal of Advanced Nursing,* 25: 36–44.

McClure, L. (1993) Care in the community, an anthropological enquiry into the experiences of informal male carers living in Creston, a small housing estate in central England. Unpublished MSc Thesis.

Morris, J. (1993) *Independent lives? Community care and disabled people.* London: Macmillan.

Morton, A. and Mackenzie, A. (1994) An exploratory study of the consumers' views of carer support groups. *Journal of Clinical Nursing,* 3: 63–4.

Neale, B. (1993) Informal care and community care. In: Clarke, D. *The future of palliative care.* Milton Keynes: Open University Press.

Nolan, M. and Grant, G. (1989) Addressing the needs of informal carers: a neglected area of nursing practice. *Journal of Advanced Nursing,* 14: 950–61.

Nolan, M., Grant, G. and Keady, J. (1996) *Understanding family care.* Buckingham: Open University Press.

Nolan, M., Grant, G. and Keady, J. (1999) Supporting family carers: a facilitative model for community nursing practice. In: McIntosh, J. *Research issues in community nursing.* London: Macmillan.

Norman, A. (1985) *Triple jeopardy: growing old in a second homeland.* London: Centre for Policy on Ageing.

Nuttall, S.R. (1992) *Financing long term care in Britain.* London: Institute of Actuaries.

Office for National Statistics (1998) *Informal carers.* London: OPCS.

Ong, B. (1991) Researching need in district nursing. *Journal of Advanced Nursing,* 16: 638–47.

Parker, G. (1990) *With due care and attention, a review of research on informal care* (second edition). London: Family Policy Studies Centre.

Parker, G. (1993) *With this body: caring and disability in marriage.* Milton Keynes: Open University Press.

Richardson, R. (1998) Taken for granted. In: Fish, D. and Coles, C. *Developing professional judgement in health care: learning through the critical appreciation of practice.* Oxford: Butterworth/Heineman.

Smith, P. (1992) *The emotional labour of nursing.* London: Macmillan.

Tinson, S. (1995) Assessing health need: a community perspective. In: Cain, P., Hyde, V. and Howkins, E. (eds) *Community nursing: dimensions and dilemmas.* London: Arnold.

Twigg, J. (1989) Models of carers: how do social care agencies conceptualise their relationships with informal carers. *Journal of Social Policy,* 18: 53–66.

Twigg, J. (1992) Personal care and the interface between the district nursing and home help services. In: Davies, B., Bebbington, A. and Charnely, H. (eds) *Resources, needs and outcomes in community based care.* Aldershot: Gower.

United Kingdom Central Council for Nursing, Midwifery and Health Visiting (UKCC). (1992) *Professional code of conduct.* London: UKCC.

United Kingdom Central Council for Nursing, Midwifery and Health Visiting (UKCC). (1994) *The future of professional practice. The Council's standards for education and practice following registration.* London: UKCC.

Ungerson, C. (1987) *Policy is personal.* London: Tavistock.

Versluysen, M. (1980) Old wives tales? Women healers in English history. In: Davies, C. (ed.) *Rewriting nursing history.* London: Croom Helm.

Walker, A. (1996) *Young carers and their families.* London: Office for National Statistics.

Weightman, G. (19990 *A real break. Guidebook on the provision of short-term breaks.* London: Crown Copyright (14993 PPD 5k IP).

Whyte, D.A. (1997) *Explanations in family nursing.* London: Routledge.

Wilkin, D. (1979) Caring for the mentally handicapped child. London: Croom Helm.

Care management and community nursing

6

Paul Swift and David Pontin

Introduction

The impact of the NHS and Community Care Act (1990) has been wide and far-reaching for both clients and care workers. Yet little research has been carried out into the changes to the everyday working practices of community nurses and the effect this has had on other aspects of their work and role. This chapter is an attempt to redress this situation. We report on research that investigates community nurses' experiences of acting as care managers and relate our findings to the literature on care management.

The research project took place in the county of Somerset, England, during the summer and autumn of 1999. It was part of a larger project investigating the impact of care management on the professional identity of practitioners. The work reported on here concerns a purposive sample of seven community nurses who function as care managers. They were approached to participate in the study and in-depth, semi-structured interviews were carried out with them in their work base. The interviews were audiotaped, transcribed and analysed for latent meaning. The seven 'G' grade community nurses all performed community nursing work in addition to their care management responsibilities – five were district nursing team leaders and two specialized in disability issues.

In order to place the present work in context, the chapter begins by providing an overview of issues pertinent to care management in the UK. It then shows how the Somerset model of care management addresses some of those issues, in particular, role boundaries and access to budgets. The findings from the research interviews are then presented in terms of the 'added value of care management', 'professional tribalism', 'training the next generation' and 'commissioning for individuals'. The chapter concludes by highlighting the implications for primary care groups (PCGs) and primary care trusts (PCTs).

Emerging issues

The principles underpinning the introduction of care management in welfare are inextricably linked in the UK to the development of 'care in the community'. This is a term which refers to the range of services used to support people with health and social care needs to live in non-institutional settings. The phrase was coined in the late 1950s specifically to describe alternatives to long-term care for people with health problems and those with learning disabilities, in response to a series of reports and publications which brought to public attention the poor standard of Britain's mental hospitals (Goffman, 1961; DHSS, 1971, 1979). During the 1960s and 1970s the rate of new admissions to institutional care for these client groups fell as both the NHS and the newly created social services departments began to develop a network of community services which allowed people either to remain in their own homes or in supported accommodation. It was not until the 1980s that an accelerated programme of hospital closures began, as evidence emerged that care in the community might prove a less expensive option (Renshaw et al., 1988).

The closure programme marked a real shift in the balance of welfare provision as social models of disability were used to challenge the appropriateness of medical regimes for people whose primary needs were not health-related. Yet the costs of caring for these two groups had remained relatively stable as a proportion of the total welfare budget. The real problem for a Conservative government committed to controlling public expenditure was the rapid growth in the numbers of people surviving into so-called 'old-old age' (beyond 85 years). The 'demographic challenge' to advanced industrialized societies of increased longevity lay in the desire to reconcile traditions of cradle-to-grave provision of health and social care with slow economic growth and rising costs of care (Coleman, 1995; Lewis and Glennester, 1996). As Davies (1995a) points out, irrespective of their systems for financing health and social care, a trend towards care in the community could be traced across northern Europe, the USA and Australasia.

The reform to care programmes for elderly people in Australia in the mid-1980s was sparked by an unplanned and unco-ordinated expansion of publicly funded nursing home beds. These were characterized by poor assessment procedures, lack of rehabilitative care, inadequate co-ordination between agencies and inefficient financial systems that favoured the use of institutional care. The reforms provided funds for more home care services paid from central funds. They created a system for gatekeeping admission to residential and nursing homes through geriatric assessment teams, and more recent community options programmes have enhanced the role of holistic assessments in the process (Davies, 1995a). Across Scandinavia, home and community care schemes have been established, where responsibility for housing, social care and health care have been devolved to the lowest tier of local government, and health and social care professionals have been encouraged to work together more effectively (Coleman, 1995; Davies, 1995a). In the Netherlands, care 'mediators' carry personal care budgets and assessments of need are carried out by a range of staff (including nurses) and decision-making about care packages is delegated to multi-disciplinary committees (Evers, 1995).

In the UK, the publication of an Audit Commission report in 1986, drew attention to the dramatic consequences of the easy availability of special social security payments for beds in private residential and nursing homes to anyone qualifying on grounds of income and savings, irrespective of their need for a particular type of care. This 'perverse incentive', which had cost a mere £10 million in 1979, was predicted to account for £1 billion-worth of welfare expenditure by the end of the decade. In response, the Secretary of State for Health and Social Security invited Sir Roy Griffiths, Chief Executive of one of the country's leading supermarket chains, to review how public funds were used to support community care policy and to advise the government on options for using those funds more effectively.

The style and content of the review was highly symbolic. It reflected the reforming zeal of the Prime Minister's financial management initiative (PM, 1984) which obliged government departments to demonstrate the most effective, efficient and economic means of delivering public services. Also, the appointment of a captain of the retailing sector of industry signalled the government's determination to introduce market disciplines and practices into the delivery of health and social care. The government's avowed intention was to reduce local authorities' influence over welfare by splitting off the role of purchasing or commissioning services from the role of providing them. The American experience of 'case' or 'care management', already trialled in the Kent Care Scheme, offered the practical means to the ideological end of disaggregating state-funded welfare provision by assessing needs and purchasing care on an individual basis.

Care management: the cornerstone of community care

Sir Roy Griffiths' findings (Griffiths, 1988) were largely accepted by the government and put into effect in the 1990 NHS and Community Care Act. A major disappointment for the government was Sir Roy's failure to find alternatives to the traditional role of social services in assessing and arranging care for clients, although the issue was debated publicly. In their responses to the White Paper preceding the Act, some members of the medical community argued for locating care management in primary health care settings. General practitioners (GPs) could then co-ordinate assessments of care needs which would consolidate the referral process into a local, accessible resource that already represented a major case-finding source for social services. The argument claimed that this made good sense because GPs tend to know of the needs of both patients and their carers (Maclean, 1989), patients place a high degree of trust in GPs compared to other caring professions and they are more likely to turn to them at times of crisis (Hardy et al., 1996). Indeed, Griffiths (1988) declared himself 'struck by differences between arrangements for provision of medical and non-medical care', concluding that 'it would be too elaborate and inappropriate for a similar system to be set up for non-medical care' (p. iv). Giving GPs a pivotal role in care management would therefore confirm the 'natural order' of team working within health care settings and, if the views of NHS general managers were to be believed, would accord with GPs' desire to protect themselves from being 'managed' (Maclean, 1989).

These arguments were a foretaste of the more recent debate surrounding PCGs. However, the crucial difference was that although PCGs go to the heart of the GPs' remit and their contractual relationship with the NHS, most GPs regard community care as peripheral to their role as medical practitioners (a view unanimously confirmed by our nurse respondents). This lack of enthusiasm on the part of GPs limited Sir Roy Griffiths' (1988) ambitions for them to 'ensure that local social services authorities are aware of their patients' needs for non-health care' (para 1.6.2), whereas the White Paper hoped that 'local arrangements to enable individual GPs to make their full contribution to community care' (para 4.13) might transform relationships between GPs and social services departments hitherto characterized by 'considerable mutual misunderstanding and even mistrust' (Hardy *et al.*, 1996: 162). A space had opened into which community nurses might tread.

Although local government was able to retain its role in purchasing services through a system of care management, the provider functions of the local state would be reorganized so as to be functionally separate – what became known as the 'purchaser/provider split'. The 1990 Act places upon local authorities a formal obligation to assess an individual's need for community care services, to make plans and purchase services to meet those needs through a designated 'care manager'. This process of care management was designed to be 'the cornerstone of high quality care' in the community (para 1.1). Griffiths (1988) was keen to emphasize that the role of care manager might be taken on by people from a range of occupational backgrounds. In most cases it was likely to be either a social worker, a community nurse or an occupational therapist. However, whichever professional group care managers were drawn from, they would be expected to use the expertise and experience of others in accomplishing the tasks associated with care management:

First is the initial assessment of need involving service user, carer and other professionals, who reach agreement, with the care manager, on how needs will be met. Second is the drawing up of a plan, also agreed by all parties. Third is the negotiation of agreements, or contracts, with organisations providing the required services. Fourth is the monitoring of the plan through regular case reviews to ascertain whether the agreed services are having the desired effect and, if not, to see how far the person's needs may have changed and require different services.

(SSI, 1991)

As lead agency in community care, most local authorities decided either to add care management to the existing repertoire of tasks undertaken by their social care staff, or to designate a new class of employees as *care managers*. In the latter, the post of care manager is generally open to applicants with a range of health or social care qualifications and occasionally people with relevant experience but no professional qualifications. Some 'have sought to establish care management as equal to, but different from social work'

(Ogden, 1994: 101), employing care managers on the same pay scales, with the same career structure and the same supervision as social workers. A survey of care management arrangements carried out in 1997 found that a third of all authorities used health staff to co-ordinate *assessments* of need (SSI/PSSRU, 1998a) and noted that 'at the more inclusive end of the spectrum, district nurses, hospital discharge co-ordinators and specialist nurses could and did undertake the full range of care management tasks' (SSI/PSSRU, 1998b). It concluded that the most effective practice was to be found where there were strong organizational links between primary care workers and those responsible for the care management process. Such linkages, it claimed, ensured that 'a more holistic view of the individual user and his or her situation' would be gained (SSI/PSSRU, 1998b).

Some early experimental care management schemes located social workers/ care managers in primary health care settings. It was found that poor referral rates from their health colleagues reflected 'considerable uncertainty about what care management meant, even among the care managers themselves' (Harrison and Thistlethwaite, 1993: 75), whereas negative perceptions of each others' role proved a major impediment to successful joint working across the health/social services boundary. Other studies confirmed the importance of organizational arrangements that clearly demarcate the roles and responsibilities of those involved in one of three ways. These arrangements involved either the 'co-location' of staff in a single workplace, or 'attachments' of named social services workers to primary health care teams, or by 'awareness raising' to ensure that primary health care workers know when, how and who to contact about issues relating to care management. Such arrangements can lead to more efficient and better quality assessments of needs and a more effective allocation of resources. Hardy *et al.* (1996: 176) found the co-location model to be popular with the staff involved in their study as it led to improved response times for requests for help and a reduction in professional stereotyping and mutual suspicion. Similarly, a project in Greenwich reported a surge in referrals that were dealt with successfully by practice-based care managers and improvements in communication and professional co-operation, leading to 'greater satisfaction for everyone involved' (Hodgson, 1998: 89).

The Somerset model

Somerset social services department took the view that it was 'better to build on existing practice and working links, modifying arrangements where necessary and integrating the principles of assessment and care management into every day work' (SSSD, 1991). This led to an approximate division of labour within community care whereby a social worker would co-ordinate the assessment and management of care where a person's needs were primarily of a social nature. Specially trained nurse assessors based within primary health care teams would take on these tasks where the needs were primarily for nursing care. Having assessed a client's needs, the nurse assessors may draw on the social service budget to arrange nursing home placements or to arrange health, rehabilitation and social care packages delivered in the client's home. There is an expectation that nurses and social workers will work together in all cases. This means that as a matter of policy, care plans have to be jointly agreed before the funding for care may be released. It is important to note here that the remit of nurse assessors is determined by their function as a nurse. When they take on the care management role, nurse sssessors take on responsibility for ensuring that colleagues have completed their assessment tasks, that care plans have been implemented satisfactorily and that reviews are carried out at the correct time.

THE ADDED VALUE OF CARE MANAGEMENT

The nurse assessors in Somerset are employed as 'G' grade district nursing team leaders and are experienced practitioners. Many of the skills they identified as being essential to their role as care managers had been developed through their nursing careers, although none felt that their professional training had prepared them for the specific tasks of care management. All agreed that the joint training programme for health and social services care managers designed by the social services department had been useful in providing basic knowledge about community care law, benefits regulations and local service provision. Existing skills had been developed to include assessment of the social element of clients' care needs while their nursing knowledge was sometimes used in new ways, for example, giving advice to staff in nursing homes on the care required by clients they had placed.

The nurse assessors stressed the importance of communication in the role of care manager since much of the work is taken up with co-ordinating the professional effort of others, either at the stage of assessing needs or when arranging services to meet those needs. Their experience as team managers and their seniority within primary health care teams helped in this respect and gave them the confidence to deal not just with the usual range of health and social services staff, but also with environmental health officers and housing officers. In this respect, the nurses' jobs had been enhanced by taking on the care management role; indeed, they regarded it to some extent as a positive extension of what they had always been doing. They took particular satisfaction from being able to involve themselves more fully in their clients' lives and felt they had achieved greater control over the outcomes they could achieve for them:

> It's made the job more interesting. It's given me a lot more responsibility and it's also nice to see people right through to the end and then when they do become very ill you still go and see them in the nursing home, you're still a part of their family.

Some went so far as to suggest that their practice now resembled that of their social work colleagues in its emphasis upon holistic assessments and a concern for all aspects of a client's caring needs:

We obviously have got clinical skills and we are able to do that; that is the focus we are coming from, not maybe so much of the social care. But because a lot of work now is tied up with multi-agency working and supporting people in a number of different environments, we have to be very much more aware of the infrastructure and the net that keeps people going outside.

A specialist disability nurse commented that by spending so much of her working life with social workers, she could not help but be assimilated into their occupational culture. The influence upon her professional practice has been a broadening of her assessment repertoire to encompass a consideration of not just health needs but also the role of carers, the impact of stress on clients and carers, the underwriting of care costs and the benefits of working flexibly with other agencies. Yet reciprocal professional influences also flowed in the other direction:

I see social workers being much more clued up now about the medical conditions of the people they are working with.

A potential downside of the care management role is a reduction in the opportunities for direct practice, with all the nurse assessors reporting a withdrawal from some of the practical tasks of nursing. This reflected, in part, their seniority within the profession, the consequent demands of nurse management and the trend of downward delegation of tasks to health care assistants/auxiliaries and non-nursing carers. The need for clinical skills remains and some argue that the 'delivery of more intensive and high technology nursing care in the home means that community nurses will also need to *develop* their clinical skills, whether or not they are providing the care directly' (Kirk and Glendenning, 1998: 377) [emphasis added]. Most of the nurse assessors made a conscious effort to 'keep their hand in' by carrying out a community care review while performing some routine nursing tasks. And they were surprised by how much time could be taken up just dealing with one care-managed client, much of it spent on the telephone arranging services or liaising with other professionals. One felt it necessary to explain to her team why she appeared to be doing less direct work than before because:

. . . that helps to eliminate resentment when people think 'she's not doing anything, she just sits in the office' or 'she's just on the phone all the time'. And I think time is the biggest thing. You can spend practically all day on one case sorting things out and sometimes you do come away at the end of the day thinking, 'what have I done, what on earth have I spent a whole day doing?' Whereas the 'old-fashioned way', if you like, the way we used to work, was much more, was 'yeah, I've done all of that work', but it was very task-oriented really, and was that really the best use of our time? The rest of the team can probably fulfil that for less money and at the end of the day if it gets the patient home or the care they need, then it is worthwhile.

But it is the nature of the relationship between the nurse assessors and their clientèle that has undergone the most significant changes since the implementation of the community care reforms. The relationship is now predicated in notions of brokerage, advocacy and consultation. The nurse's task is not just to diagnose what care is required but also to provide options for clients to choose how it will be delivered. Care management is therefore a factor in what Kirk and Glendenning (1998) describe as the reformulation of the client's role in community nursing from patienthood to partnership. Social workers recognize this process as one of empowerment, whereby clients are encouraged and helped to take control over their own lives. That increased participation in decision-making may stimulate therapeutic effects of improved well-being, health and even mortality rates for older people being discharged from hospital (Abramson, 1990). This suggests that strategies for empowerment may also have a pragmatic rationale, where responsibilities for providing direct care fall to informal and family carers. But such a determined pursuit of choice introduces risk as a factor in the care management task.

Factors that may need to be taken into account by care managers include risks to the client of physical abuse, financial exploitation, self-harm or self-neglect. But there are also physical and emotional risks to carers who may be asked to take on a burden of caring. In some instances the impact upon the local community may also need to be taken into account. An example may be where an individual's behaviour can be bizarre or threatening. At the heart of any risk assessment there will be consideration of the relationship between clients and their carers and the identification of potential sources of conflict. This may be where the needs of clients and carers differ, or where clients and carers disagree about what is best for the client. This raises several ethical issues for care managers: what should their role be in mediating the relationship between client and carer? How far should they seek to influence and persuade clients and carers to accept their professional judgement about the best courses of action? And, how far should they go in denying a client's desire for *dependency* rather than independence? (Stevenson and Parsloe, 1993: 19). The following extracts are examples of the many case studies cited by the nurse assessors:

The gentleman who was supposed to be coming out tomorrow really needs to be going into a nursing home and I know that the situation is not going to work out, but we have to give him that chance to try at home. He has to know the risks that he is putting himself at and his wife at. We've sat down and I've spoken to his wife at home and I've spoken to him on his own, I've spoken to them both together and he knows he's at risk. He wants to take that risk because he wants to try and if it doesn't work he will be quite happy to go in somewhere. You've got to give people the chance and you have to take a calculated risk, as long as they can make an informed choice and are aware of all the options.

We had a patient recently who was at a local hospital. He was assessed and his wife couldn't cope with him at home and he'd had two MIs in quick succession, then followed by quite a severe CVA. His wife couldn't cope with him at home so it was assessed that he might require some nursing home care, so he was admitted to a local nursing home . . . We always set it up that we do a review after a patient has been in a nursing home for four weeks and when I went with the social worker (we try to do a joint first visit), he'd done remarkably well and his whole frame of mind was so different, he was really keen, really motivated and he wanted to aim for home, which his wife was absolutely staggered about because she had not heard him say this before . . . We have a rehabilitation service that has just started and, with a bit of persuasion, I was able to access the rehabilitation service who are now going into him every day in the nursing home so that we could set up a plan of care for six weeks with intense physiotherapy to see if we could actually aim for home. He's been home, we've tried wheelchairs round and the wife is now really quite keen as well on getting him back which, if he had just gone into the home and been left, I don't think he would have an opportunity to see if he could fulfil his potential. We're in the middle of this and it was only about two and half weeks ago we set up the outreach service, so it's still early days and we won't know if he can actually go home. But at least he can know that he tried his utmost, and his wife as well.

I can recall a lady who went home to live with her husband and we all had doubts about how well it would work, but they were so devoted to each other and so determined to make it work that the heart in us said this lady has got to go home while the head was saying it's not the right place for her. Fortunately, everything has worked out very well and this lady has been at home with her husband for over two years now. There have been no problems with the care package at all. You just feel that their quality of life as a couple has been so much better. They don't put their hands up and say, 'we were right all along', because those of us who were involved wanted them to have what they wanted. It's the difficulty between the person and the profession – the professional in you says there are certain risk factors here, this is what we think might be a problem. But the personal part of you thinks, 'I so want this lady to go home because from the psychological point of view she is going to be happier and her husband is going to be happier'. It worked, so we were very pleased to put our hands up and say we were wrong . . . it's better now and I think the fact that the caring professions' attitude has changed so that we give people the choice now. We can say, 'these are the options' and they decide what's going to be best for them. And if you don't agree with it, you have to respect the fact that it's their wish and that you've got to do your best for them. As long as they are aware of the reservations you have and why, at the end of the day it is their decision.

The proper role of the nurse assessor as care manager might best be described as that of risk assessor, facilitator and, ultimately, client advocate. The idea that nurses act as advocates for their clients, that is, they act as representatives for, and act in the best interests of, their patients, has surfaced at various times in the past and has been part of the 'professionalisation project' of nursing since the mid-1970s (Christman, 1976; MacKay and Ault, 1977; Smith, 1977; Booth, 1995; Davies, 1995b; Neal, 1995; Wright, 1995). In particular, it has formed a major element of the development of 'new nursing' (Salvage, 1990). The argument for nurses acting as advocates for their patients within the health care system was based on the continuity of the relationship between nurses and their clients, and nurses' close social proximity to their patients in class terms. However, there have been problems in confirming this notion due to a discrepancy between professional rhetoric and nurses' priorities and their inclinations when it comes to action. Buckenham and McGrath (1984) attempted to interpret the everyday social interactions in health care settings from the nurses' perspectives by use of a critical incident technique. Nurses were given a choice between acting as a patient's advocate or as a bureaucratic agent in hypothetical situations. The majority of those involved in the study chose the bureaucratic agent role. They only acted as patient advocate when their membership of the health care team was not compromised. The explanation given by Buckenham and McGrath (1984) is that the primary affiliation of nursing staff is to the health care team, not to their patients.

The examples cited here illustrate the different responses to situations between the nurse assessors and the nurses in the study by Buckenham and McGrath (1984). The extension of the community nursing role to include brokerage, risk assessment, facilitation of care and consultation appears to reinforce the likelihood of them acting as client advocates. This may also be due to the separation made between purchasing care and providing it directly, and merits further investigation

All the nurse assessors emphasized the importance of communication skills in the role of care manager. Several mentioned diplomacy and the art of not 'treading on the toes' of other professionals providing a service to the nurse assessor's care-managed clients. In most cases a clear demarcation of professional roles and skills means that this is not a problem. However, in Somerset the fact that nurse assessors are managing some of the care provided by nursing homes can lead to potentially difficult situations:

Going into nursing homes has opened up a completely new area because before we never ever went into nursing homes. At the beginning it was very awkward and it's taken probably a couple of years into community care for them to feel happy with us because some of the matrons felt a bit threatened ... Maybe it was a little bit because we were nurses and I suppose professionally we were questioning the care, which is a little bit unnerving. It was down to building relationships and them getting to know our role, that we weren't there as watchdogs and we were there just in the interests of the patients. It works really well now and there's nothing left of that, but at the beginning you definitely got vibes when you walked through the door.

There was another side to this relationship with nursing homes. Many of the problems which arise for residents in nursing homes seem to occur within a few months of their arrival and can be sorted out quite easily by the resident or their relatives without recourse to the nurse assessor. Sometimes the client or a relative will contact the nurse assessor first concerning a query about the care that is being delivered in a nursing home. Because of their nursing background, nurse assessors are often able to explain that the care is appropriate or will allay fears by contacting the home on their behalf:

You're the unbiased person. You're there as their representative . . . They might say 'They've not done anything about my teeth, I haven't been to see an optician, I'm left in bed till lunchtime'. You can negotiate with the staff to see why this is happening, you can try and improve the situation.

PROFESSIONAL TRIBALISM

Perhaps a more far-reaching consequence of these changes in Somerset is the reduction in what Dalley (1989) terms 'professional tribalism'. Besides including community nurses in care management and providing joint training for social workers and nurses in assessment and commissioning, Somerset Social Services now operates a system of GP attachment for all social services social workers. A project to pilot the system aimed to improve liaison between social workers, GPs and community nurses during the assessment and delivery of community care services to older people.

This raises questions about boundaries that practitioners perceive between their respective professional groupings in Somerset given the different working arrangements there. The specialist disability nurse identified two boundaries between social workers and nurses: the first concerning the use of professional language, the second referred to budgets. The first boundary entails the use of language to define what is to be included and what is to be excluded from the particular field of work. In the past, joint working has been bedevilled by a kind of negative turf war or passing the buck, where one group attempts to deny responsibility for meeting the needs of individuals or groups of clients. This game is played out where professional responsibility or remit merges with political power in the form of agencies that act to protect their budgets from outside 'interference'. The budgetary issue in Somerset has been addressed in part by an agreement to allocate a 'call-off' budget made up of social service monies for use by Trust personnel to purchase nursing care. However, the specialist disability nurse pointed to the plight of people with learning disabilities who suffer strokes and are shunted between services until agreement is reached about accepting responsibility for their care needs. She remained sanguine, commenting that 'the seamless service may not exist when it comes to money, but it can exist when people work together'.

A major benefit of the close working relationship is that when things go wrong, all sides work together to seek a solution rather than trying to lay the blame on others. The ethic of pursuing a 'needs-led' service was apparent in their responses:

> Over the years the demands on us for nurse-specific interventions has increased as we have shed the personal care component that has been handed over to social services. So, to be asked suddenly to take it on for even a short period causes us problems. But, there are means and ways of getting round it and there are various budgetary avenues we can go down to meet that crisis. So, whilst it is causing conflict, it is only thanks to the good partnership between us and social services that we can discuss it, debate it and find ways and means of getting round it: we may engage agency staff to cover the crisis. We negotiate and we try and make it seamless, but we accept that sometimes there will be gaps. So it causes conflict, it causes difficulty, but it can be overcome ... We had this situation about a fortnight ago where [social worker] was struggling to try and provide cover and it wasn't easy, but we negotiated, we compromised and co-operated as best we could. The service provision wasn't perhaps quite what the individuals hoped it would be, but then it was needs *met* rather than what was *wanted*.

The most experienced of the nurses recalled what little contact she had with social workers prior to community care. Previously, if a patient was deemed to require some form of residential care they would be referred by letter to the local social services team and the nurses had no direct contact with the social worker who took on the case. She summed up the benefits of the new working relationship as, 'better communication, better use of resources, better delivery of care, swifter assessment'.

The nurses had little doubt that the most important factor in generating that good working relationship was the joint training initiated by the local authority and health trust in the run up to implementation of community care in April 1993. Training modules were designed to bring nursing and social service staff together so that they could not only learn about their obligations under the new legislation, but also understand more about each other's ways of approaching the tasks associated with community care.

That GPs have a poor understanding of how community care works in practice was ascribed by the nurses to unwillingness to invest time in something peripheral to their day-to-day work. Whatever their reluctance to become involved in the early days of community care (and invitations to GPs to attend the joint training sessions were rarely taken up) the very success of the nurse assessor scheme means that GPs have overwhelming confidence in the nurses' abilities to pursue successful outcomes for their patients. Indeed, a detectable trend in primary care has been the delegation by GPs of a 'considerable proportion of their workload' to practice nurses, community nurses and health visitors (Jenkins-Clarke *et al.*, 1998). Some GPs apparently do act as though the community care reforms had never taken place – promising patients inappropriate care or asking the nurses to arrange care without a proper assessment – but the nurses regard this as an indication of ignorance about the system rather than a deliberate attempt to undermine them.

One of the by-products of the Somerset system is that nurses have been empowered to challenge these assumptions about the appropriateness of ongoing care not just amongst GPs but also among hospital doctors and even consultants. There is some evidence that the presence of community colleagues can alter the attitude of ward nursing staff in favour of greater autonomy for patients in decision-making. This can help speed up the discharge process which is an important consideration for Trusts anxious to reduce the incidence of 'bed-blocking' (Carter and MacInnes, 1996):

There are instances where I'm asked to go and assess somebody in hospital say, and they haven't actually reached their peak. Say they'd had a stroke and they were still being rehabilitated and they are asking me to do an assessment for nursing home care – well, at that time, yes, they might need nursing home care, but two months down the line they could probably manage in residential care. So you have to look also at the long-term and I've actually asked GPs to delay discharge for a month just to see how somebody can do after intensive physiotherapy and occupational therapy. If you've got a valid point, yes they will listen. (Would you have had that sort of clout in the past?) No, no. It comes with care in the community and with experience.

. . . the number of times you go to a ward and they are wanting to come home and the ward staff are saying, 'Well, there's no way this person can go home'. We are saying that is their choice, that is their right; it may be risky and we may professionally think it is not the right thing to do. And that can be difficult at times, but if it is their burning ambition to go home, then we can look together at putting together appropriate care packages to support them. That doesn't always work because resources are finite and if somebody is incredibly vulnerable, you may not be able to put in the right level of care in to make them safe. But, providing they have got relatively all their marbles, that is their choice. Providing you can go through the risk assessments with them and their carers and do all you can do to minimalize the risks then I think people should be entitled to do that.

The nurse assessors are now recognized as an expert resource within GPs surgeries in Somerset – community care is seen as part of their remit whether they become care manager or not because of their close links with social work colleagues. This set of relationships has interesting implications as we move towards PCGs; indeed, one of the nurse assessors is a PCG Board member:

I see myself really as a member of this team which is the day-to-day area that we work in, so it's a clinical primary care setting. That has altered: a few years ago there was far more contact between our [district nurse] colleagues elsewhere, but because of the evolution of primary care working we've become much more focused into primary health care teams. I don't think it is there by a long shot yet, but that is where we are going. So we actually identify more with the surgeries even though we are not employed by the GPs – we are employed by a Trust – we are autonomous, we work to this caseload. Our work is generated by this practice, but basically we are very autonomous in the way that we work.

TRAINING THE NEXT GENERATION

Several of the nurse assessors regularly facilitate students as practice teachers and all host student placements in their teams. They acknowledged the increasing emphasis in nurse training upon research-based practice, the management of care as well as a positive willingness to shed some of the tasks traditionally associated with nursing. Their commentary on the changing nature of nursing and nurse training within the context of the expansion of both the primary health and community care sectors reflected themes of partnership, team working, flexibility and delegation:

Prior to 1993, district nurses were taking total responsibility for care. After that there was the division of care responsibilities between nursing and personal care and nurses were reluctant to let go and they felt that only they could do it, only they had the skill to look after somebody totally. I think what we have learned is that others can do some of our jobs just as well. Other colleagues will probably condemn me for saying this, but most professional carers can do some of our caring tasks competently, adequately and to a set standard – not everybody. What I have learned is that we can work in co-operation and partnership and achieve what we set out to achieve, it can be done.

COMMISSIONING FOR INDIVIDUALS

Our presentation of the findings from the research lead us now to pose the questions, 'What is the future for the role of community nurses in care management?' and 'What lessons can be learned from the Somerset approach?'. Rummery's (1998) model of 'commissioning for individuals' proposes that rather than commission different or distinctly new forms of service for clients, commissioners should concentrate on improving client access to the existing provision which is supplied by social services or other contracted care agencies. Within such schemes it may be that primary health care team members may carry out some or all of the assessment and other functions of care management. Alternatively, individuals may be employed by the primary health care team to fulfil the care manager function or, as Lankshear et al. (1999)

describe, a social service care manager may be placed with a primary health care team to improve access for clients. What is of note here in this model is that it maintains the status quo as far as forms of service provision are concerned. There is limited opportunity to change the range and nature of services which may be offered so co-operative working and collaborative practice are essential for this to be successful in meeting client needs and reducing the number of inappropriate assessment visits by health and social care professionals. However, while there may be collaboration and co-operation between health and social care professionals who have a remit for commissioning, there may be little opportunity for inter-professional working for those front-line staff who do not.

In describing her work, Rummery (1998) points out that models of commissioning provided those involved with the means of finding out about the remit of their peers in other agencies. For those people who took the opportunity offered to them, they reported a decrease in the 'professional tribalism' because the greater understanding led to more effective and efficient communication which, in turn, led to a reduction in delays in organising services. Although the 'commissioning for individuals' model provided the greatest opportunity for inter-agency worker collaboration, a major problem with it was the few openings available for strategic commissioning or service development.

One way of overcoming this problem is suggested in the *The New NHS – Modern and Dependable* (DOH, 1997) and possibly strengthens the case for involving nurses in community care commissioning as in Somerset. PCGs will have to, 'bring together GPs and community nurses in each area to work together to improve the health of local people [to] better integrate primary and community health services and work more closely with social services on both planning and delivery' (DOH, 1997: 33–4).

Besides these strategic considerations, the workload of care management undertaken by nurse assessors provides significant relief to social service staff because as many as 20% of care packages in recent years have been wholly or jointly managed by nurse assessors. The implications of the enhanced role of these community nurses in Somerset goes further in the way it addresses the problem of 'artificial boundaries' thrown up by the challenge of people who have a complex combination of health and social needs which do not match the configuration of services commissioned by health and social care commissioners (Twigg, 1997). Providing community nurses access to their budgets for commissioning social care services may be seen as one way of attempting to ensure that 'seamless' social and health care may be provided to clients (Rummery, 1998).

There are a number of benefits that may arise from co-ordinating services in this way. These include having a system to ensure that vulnerable, high-risk clients are not overlooked by health or social services because they are considered to be another agency's responsibility. There may also be a reduction in the number of hospital beds that are occupied for prolonged periods and therefore 'unavailable' to the system. Alternatively, there may also be reductions in the emergency admission of clients to hospital, due to crises in home or social care arrangements, where there is little agreement over who has responsibility for assessing and commissioning services.

These benefits seem to be present in the Somerset context if we examine some of the clinical indicators issued by the NHS Executive for the south-west peninsula for emergency re-admission rates (NHS Executive, 1999). Over the three-year period in which data is presented by the NHS Executive, only Somerset achieves positive movement on all three indicators. There is year-on-year variation between and within the health authority scores on these indicators so caution must be exercised in interpreting the data and it is likely that additional factors will have influenced the scores. However, during the period when the community nurses in Somerset were assessing client need and commissioning community care services, the emergency re-admission rate to hospital decreased, the rate of discharge within 56 days for people with strokes increased as did the discharge rate for people sustaining hip fractures. Although these indicators do not provide conclusive evidence that the community care assessment and commissioning arrangements directly led to these outcomes they do provide useful pointers which add to the argument for including nurses in community care management in this way.

Conclusion

The research into the Somerset model reported on here raises a number of interesting issues for community nursing which warrant further examination and investigation. First, nurses describe how they transfer their existing skills, such as assessment, care planning and inter-personal communication, to the role of care manager. However, they refine and adapt them as well as developing new skills when addressing care management issues. Many of the nurse assessors view the care manager role as a positive extension to their current practice and begin to conceptualize the practice of community nursing differently. They describe the ways in which the nurse assessor role allows them to practise in an holistic way which corresponds to the ideal of community nursing but is different to their actual, previous experience of the work. Further research work is required to map out the circumstances which encourage the development of these skills and the consequences for 'usual' community nursing of this reconceptualization. Such work will assist educators to identify ways in which training programmes for future community nurses may be adapted to include the development of these new skills. Also, there is the possibility for developing new and innovative ways of delivering the 'usual' service.

A consequence of the nurse assessor role is a reduction in the amount of direct patient care carried out by community nurses who function in that capacity. The consequences of this may be seen in the change in the relationship between nurse assessors and their patients from direct caregiver to risk assessor, facilitator and client advocate. Community nurses talk about the changes they make to their own ideas of the nature of community nursing and the ways they try to manage the impressions of their community nursing team colleagues. There are striking similarities to the conundrum faced by health visitors who have to account for their practice when faced with the question 'What exactly do you do?' Additional research is required to investigate how the wider primary health care team adjusts to the change in community nursing practice when the nurse assessor is incorporated into everyday activity and how the workload of community nursing is redistributed. Questions are also raised about the degree of clinical supervision and peer support necessary for nurses to fulfil the role successfully to meet client, organizational and professional requirements for efficiency, effectiveness and safety.

Perhaps the key element of the Somerset model that seems to have had the most profound effect on the development of the nurse assessor role is the access to budgets. The ability to assess and prescribe packages of care and then maintain contact and evaluate the effectiveness of the package seems to have underwritten the development of the advocacy element of the role. Nurse assessors describe how access to budgets combined with joint training with social workers has led to an increased understanding of the roles of social care workers and the language used in the world of social care. The effect of this seems to be a decrease in professional tribalism. Further work is required to identify the influence of joint assessment training where access to budgets is not available.

One consequence of a care management system which encourages community nurses to play a positive role in discharge planning and to empower clients by giving them choice, is that it is likely to make the discharge process more efficient. This, in turn, is likely to have an economic consequence for health care trusts that provide acute care. Further work is required to quantify the degree of efficiency and identify the potential cost savings to the public exchequer.

Finally, we come to the effect of the nurse assessor role on the development and functioning of PCGs/PCTs. GPs rely heavily upon community nurses in Somerset both to foster relationships between primary health care teams and social services departments, as well as to manage care packages for their patients. This reliance places nurses in a potentially strong position both within primary heatlh care teams and PCGs/PCTs. The GP–social worker relationship has been fraught with difficulties of finding mutually acceptable ways of working, professional stereotyping, lack of trust, and differing perspectives (Khan et al., 1998). It appears that the nurse assessors have found ways to bridge the divide between the two worlds of the primary health care teams and social care. By literally interpreting the languages of these worlds to the various participants and having the authority for action from their community nursing role and the advocacy from their access to the social services budget, nurse assessors appear to have opened up a new space for action and professional development. This space takes on greater significance when the role of nurses on PCG/PCT Boards is taken into account. There is the opportunity for nurse assessors to take the issues of care management right to the heart of PCG/PCTs via community nurse representation on executive Boards. This possibility for action needs to monitored and evaluated in comparison with areas where nurse assessors have yet to be developed.

References

Abramson, J. (1990) Enhancing patient participation: clinical strategies in the discharge planning process. *Social Work in Health Care*, 14: 970–3.

Booth, J. (1995) Advantages of primary nursing in geriatric day hospitals. *British Journal of Nursing*, 4: 467–8.

Buckenham, J. and McGrath, G. (1984) *The social reality of nursing*. Balgowlah, Australia: ADIS Health Science Press.

Carter, H. and MacInnes, P. (1996) Nursing attitudes to the care of elderly patients at risk of continuing care. *Journal of Advanced Nursing*, 24: 448–55.

Christman, L. (1976) The autonomous nursing staff in the hospital. *Nursing Administration Quarterly*, 1: 37–44.

Coleman, B. (1995) European models of long-term care in the home and community. *International Journal of Health Sciences*, 25: 455–74.

Dalley, G. (1989) Professional ideology or organizational tribalism? In: Taylor, R. and Ford, J. (eds) *Social work and health care research highlights 19*. London: Jessica Kingsley.

Davies, B. (1995a) The reform of community and long-term care of elderly persons. In: Scharf, T. and Wenger, C. *International perspectives on community care for elderly people*. Avebury: Aldershot.

Davies, C. (1995b) *Gender and the professional predicament in nursing*. Buckingham: Open University Press.

Department of Health (DOH). (1997) *The new NHS – modern and dependable*. London: HMSO.

Department of Health and Social Security (DHSS). (1971) *Better services for the mentally handicapped*. Cmnd 4683. London: HMSO.

Department of Health and Social Security (DHSS). (1979) *Report of the committee of inquiry into mental handicap nursing and care*. Cmnd 7468. London: HMSO.

Evers, A. (1995) The future of elderly care in Europe. In: Scharf, T. and Wenger, C. *International perspectives on community care for elderly people*. Avebury: Aldershot.

Goffman, E. (1961) *Asylums: essays on the social situation of mental patients and other inmates*. Harmondsworth: Penguin.

Griffiths, Sir R. (1988) *Community care: agenda for action*. London: HMSO.

Hardy, B., Leedham, I. and Wistow, G. (1996) Care manager co-location in GP practices: effects upon assessment and care management arrangements for older people. In: Bland, R. *Research highlights in social work no. 29*. London: Jessica Kingsley.

Harrison, L. and Thistlethwaite, P. (1993) Care management in a primary health care setting: pilot projects in East Sussex. In: Smith, R., Gaster, L. and Harrison, L. *et al.* (eds) *Working together for better community care*. Bristol: SAUS Publications.

Hodgeson, R. (1998) It's all good practice: linking primary care and social services in Greenwich. *Journal of Interprofessional Care*, 12: 89–91.

Jenkins-Clarke, S., Carr-Hill, R. and Dixon, P. (1998) Teams and seams: skill mix in primary care. *Journal of Advanced Nursing*, 28: 120–6.

Khan, P., Lupton, C. and Lacey, D. *et al.* (1998) Primary care groups and partnerships with social services departments: the perspectives of general practitioners. *Social Services Research*, 3: 19–28.

Kirk, S. and Glendenning, C. (1998) Trends in community care and patient participation: implications for the roles of informal carers and community nurses in the United Kingdom. *Journal of Advanced Nursing*, 28: 370–81.

Lankshear, G., Giarchi, G. and Hodges, V. (1999) The placement of a social service care manager in a GP surgery as a way to improve care access to services and improve liaison between statutory agencies. *Health and Social Care in the Community*, 7: 206–15.

Lewis, J. and Glennester, H. (1996) *Implementing the new community care*. Buckingham: Open University Press.

MacKay, C. and Ault, L. (1977) *Primary nursing: a systematic approach to individualizing nursing care*. Massachusetts: Contemporary Publishing.

Maclean, U. (1989) *Dependent territories: the frail elderly and community care*. London: London Provincial Hospitals Trust.

NHS Executive. (1999) *Quality and performance in the NHS: clinical indicators technical supplement. Annex A*. Leeds: NHS Executive.

Neal, K. (1995) Managing change: the named nurse. *Nursing Standard*, 9: 29–30.

Ogden, C. (1994) Community care – change of cosmetics? In: Davidson, R. and Hunter, S. *Community care in practice*. London: BT Batsford.

Prime Minister (PM). (1984) *Progress in financial management in government departments*. Cmnd 9297. London: HMSO.

Renshaw, J., Hampson, R. and Thomason, C. *et al.* (1988) *Care in the community: the first steps*. Aldershot: Gower.

Rummery, K. (1998) Changes in primary health care policy: the implications for joint commissioning with social services. *Health and Social Care in the Community*, 6: 429–37.

Salvage, J. (1990) The theory and practice of the 'new nursing'. *Nursing Times Occasional Paper*, 86: 42–5.

Smith, C. (1977) Primary nursing care: a substantive nursing care delivery system. *Nursing Administration Quarterly*, 1: 1–8.

Social Services Inspectorate (SSI)/Scottish Office Social Work Services Group (SOSWSG). (1991) *Care management and assessment: a practitioner's guide*. London: HMSO.

Social Services Inspectorate (SSI)/Personal Social Services Research Unit (PSSRU). (1998a) *Care management study: a report on national data*. London: DOH.

Social Services Inspectorate (SSI)/Personal Social Services Research Unit (PSSRU). (1998b) *Care management study: care management arrangements*. London: DOH.

Somerset Social Services Department (SSSD). (1991) *Report of the joint working group on assessment and care management*. Taunton: Somerset County Council.

Stevenson, O. and Parsloe, P. (1993) *Community care and empowerment*. York: Joseph Rowntree Foundation.

Twigg, J. (1997) Deconstructing the 'social bath': help with bathing at home for older and disabled people. *Journal of Social Policy*, 26: 211–32.

Wright, S. (1995) Setting a prime example. *Elderly Care*, 7: 12.

7 Covert community nursing: reciprocity in formal and informal relations

Paul Parkin

Introduction

In response to health policy changes and the development of the specialist practitioner (UKCC, 1994, 1998) during the 1990s there has been a plethora of text books covering the broader aspects of community nursing work. These texts have generally propounded a theoretical approach required for delivering health care in the community which is different from that usually applied in the more regulated hospital environment (Cain *et al.*, 1995; Twinn *et al.*, 1996; Ross and Mackenzie, 1996; Gastrell and Edwards, 1996; Burley *et al.*, 1997; Sines, 1995; Skidmore, 1997; Hennessey, 1997).

Within these broad approaches, theory has concentrated, at the macro-level, on subjects such as health policy, epidemiology, management, research, public health and health promotion and, at the micro-level, on issues such as professional/client interactions and relationships, partnership, advocacy, teamwork and collaboration. The challenge of theorizing community nursing is not disputed since, in common with many other health-related occupational groups, the professional artistry involved is 'a unique blend of know-ledge from a number of disciplines which is selectively interpreted for differing circumstances' (McIntosh, 1996). Furthermore, the number of disciplines within the umbrella term of 'community nursing' has raised questions as to its unity and, hence, to the existence of a common theoretical base (Hyde, 1995). One preeminent feature of community nursing work which complicates theory development is that principally the broad range of community nurses work in patients' homes and therefore organization within, and control of, the care environment is shared or compromised. Because of this:

> . . . a different approach is required on the part of the nurse, something perhaps only truly understood by those who know and have engaged in the work.
>
> (Hennessy and Swain 1997: 13)

This chapter aims to take up the theme of a 'different approach' by conceptualizing community nursing through a social relations model. Part of this different approach is founded on the belief that the home environment, where the majority of health care takes place, can affect the dynamics and development of the client–practitioner relationship. Within the home, many aspects of patients' social, personal and emotional lives are readily observable to community nurses who are required to take account of them within an overall programme of care. Similarly, patients and their carers can become involved with, and attached to, their regular visiting community nurses, especially if visits occur over a long period. This attachment can occur through normal social discourse and interaction. One seemingly hidden aspect of the nurse–patient relationship which is influenced directly by working in people's homes and which appears to have been given only scant cover in the theoretical literature is the existence of 'reciprocity' or social exchange. A simple definition of reciprocity refers to the equal or comparable exchange of tangible help, affection, support, advice and information between individuals and groups (Antonucci and Jackson, 1989). The norm of reciprocity is considered a powerful social force in maintaining the smooth running of everyday human relations (Gouldner, 1960) and its perceived importance can affect how individuals provide, accept and feel about forms of social exchange (Antonucci and Jackson. 1989). 'Generalized reciprocity' is customarily applied to long-term relative relationships such as between parents and children, spouses and siblings, whereas 'specific' or 'exchange reciprocity' is normally referred to shorter term, instrumentally limited relationships. Here, reciprocal acts may be confined to the giving and receiving of goods, services or affection. This chapter aims to examine the latter, specific-type reciprocity within community nurse–client relations.

It is made explicit in the nurses' code of professional conduct (UKCC, 1992) that nurses should 'refuse gifts, favours or hospitality . . . which might be interpreted as seeking to exert influence to obtain preferential consideration' yet reciprocal gift giving is frequently seen as having a vital role in maintaining effective functioning of everyday social relationships and can hold significant cultural meanings. In many respects it can also be therapeutic and to refuse a gift can be interpreted as a personal rebuff and may negatively affect the nurse–patient relationship. Judgements on the motivation and intention of the giving and receiving of gifts or hospitality is individual and hence problematic and open to wide interpretation. This may be heightened when the action takes place covertly in the patient's home and within a one-to-one interaction and may explain why research studies which explore this phenomenon can not be found. However, careful and discerning reading of much of the theoretical literature uncovers some concealed examples of reciprocity and these insights might enable this hidden practice to be built into any theory development.

This chapter will, first, provide an introductory background to set the discussion within the current policy environment of community nursing. Second, through using Weber's (1968) concepts of formal and substantive rationalism, it will argue that the hard, quantitative, 'scientific' data currently collected and analysed to plan and run an efficient service contrasts and, indeed, conflicts with the soft, affective, qualitative, 'swampy marshes' of the reality of practice (Schon, 1983) in people's homes where the main focus of work is enacted. Third, it will demonstrate the theoretical dichotomy community nurses find themselves in by contrasting the formal, professional nurse–client relations with the informal friend/confidant/carer relations which can develop through longer term, trusting relationships developed within the home environment. The focus on trust within social relations generally, and in community nurse–client relations specifically, will lead on to a discussion of reciprocity and reciprocal relations. It will discuss reciprocity as a fundamental symbol of a social relationship and draw on data which demonstrate the existence of reciprocity within community nursing practice. It will conclude that the informal, social-relations system located in the home can generate a genuine need for reciprocity and that instances of gift-giving can be legitimate and rehabilitative acts designed to promote independence and retrieve status balance within a potentially unequal relationship.

A selective policy background

Community nursing generally is increasingly being subjected to close scrutiny. Over a period of many years, but significantly during the 1970s and 1980s, there have been successive government moves to develop primary care and shift more of the population's health care into the community and into patients' and clients' homes. Historically, both financial and managerial accountability in primary care has been difficult to control. However, the need to reduce hospital costs and to promote self-responsibility for health in individuals has continued the advances. The key policy initiatives for these moves have been *Working for Patients* (DOH, 1989a), *Caring for People* (DOH, 1989b) and *The New NHS – Modern and Dependable* (DOH, 1997). The development of primary care groups (PCGs) and health improvement programmes (HImPs) has placed community nurses in the vanguard of primary health care developments and defined them as as appropriate professionals to take on lead roles (NHS Executive, 1998).

The examination of recent community nursing practice developed with the publication of the community nursing review – the Cumberlege Report (DHSS, 1986) – and was followed in 1992 by an Audit Commission report, *Homeward Bound – A New Course for Community Health* (Audit Commission, 1992). These reports criticized the community nursing service as being fragmented, illogical, underdeveloped, having high levels of variation in treatments and referrals, weak inter-agency collaboration, poor utilization of practitioners' skills and time, lack of control over caseload admissions, poor resource management and a significant lack of management information systems. Also in 1992, the Value for Money Unit produced a study on district nursing which suggested that the service was inappropriately managed, the grade and skill mix was top-heavy and work carried out by qualified district nurses could be undertaken more cost-effectively by unqualified staff.

In 1993 The NHS Management Executive (NHSME) published *New World, New Opportunities* (NHSME, 1993) which emphasized the case-management role of community nurses and predicted numerous opportunities to expand their skills and proposed major changes in roles in order to ensure survival. *Our Healthier Nation* (DOH, 1998a) has proposed community nurses' partnership skills as being a key strategy to establish 'a national contract for better health' to improve the health of all citizens.

In 1999 the Audit Commission published a follow-up national report, *First Assessment – A Review of District Nursing Services in England and Wales* (Audit Commission, 1999). This report demonstrates the enormity of the task of community nursing and the importance of being clear about service aims, financial costs and the appropriate use of time, personnel and clinical skills. The report (Audit Commission, 1999) claims that most of the professional nursing care provided in patients' homes is delivered by community nursing staff and that community nursing is 'an essential ingredient in the complex pattern of support that is needed to sustain people in their own homes' (p.15). This amounts to around 2.75 million people who are clients of the service and more than 36 million annual patient contacts costing approximately £650 million in 1997–1998. In 1996–1997, health visitors made nearly 3.7 million contacts in England alone (DOH, 1998b).

Although there is faster patient turnover and an increasing emphasis on technical, as opposed to personal, nursing care approximately half of the population aged 85 years and over are seen by a community nurse in a year and visits may occur two or three times each week. The provison of care to older people is increasing in both numbers on caseloads and in the proportion of caseloads and visits can reach a duration of several years particularly where chronic illness and the needs of the long-term sick are the foci of care (Kirk and Glendinning, 1998).

The details of these reports need not be recounted here but their substance deals principally with analysing the definition, aims, purpose and role of the service and, by implication, of community nurses themselves; yet these areas remain ill-defined (Audit Commission, 1999). Usually, the reports consider aspects of community nurses' work, such as teamwork, admission, referral and discharge criteria, quality assurance, clinical effectiveness, management and supervision, skill-mix and interprofessional relations. To some extent nurse–client relations are touched on but this is not normally their primary purpose.

Despite the extensive developments of nursing care in the community and detailed descriptions of the nature of the work, the theoretical basis of community nursing practice is poor and is under-researched (Luker and Kenrick, 1992; Bryans and McIntosh, 1986; Audit Commission, 1999).

The actual work and delivery of care by nurses in people's homes is one of the most challenging aspects to define, measure and deconstruct. Goodman (1996) suggests that there is often an assumption that community nurses' work is well-understood and that it can be easily described and defined. Although the use of cross-sectional, survey type, quantitative analyses of tasks and treatments together with frequencies and duration of visits and contacts, travelling time and 'doubles' may provide some evidence of volume and intensity of staff activity, they rely on 'rather crude activity analysis' (Goodman, 1996: 208). These are methods which Kratz (1976) found to be insufficient to study community nursing 20 years earlier and are still described as inadequate (Timmins, 1996) as they fail to capture the complexity, range and depth of health care delivered in the home. Kelly *et al.* (1998) argue that a factor constraining community nurses in their practice is the management ethos which supports a task-oriented service: 'Such a system seems to be designed to facilitate target-driven, outcome-determined, prescribed care packages'. These rational methods of quantifying care and nurses' workload means that much important work undertaken by community nurses goes unnoticed and unrecognized.

Why then are these methods of quantifying care perpetuated?

The concept of rationalism

Coles (1996) attempted to highlight the shift away from traditional views of thinking about the world by applying Weber's (1968) concept of rationalism. She argues that the achievement of goals through rational action may result in the destruction of fundamental social values. Care becomes mechanistic and non-technological work becomes devalued as it 'cannot succeed in the scientifically dominated paradigm that exists today' (Coles, 1996: 247). Key elements of prior knowledge required in community nursing include the technical, rational type of knowledge derived from the basic sciences such as pathology and physiology (MacIntosh, 1996; Bryans and McIntosh, 1996).

So, what is Weber's (1968) concept of rationalism and how is it relevant to community nursing?

Although complex and multidimensional, rationalism is central to the development of bureaucracies, which govern much of modern Western society. In essence, it describes the increasing use, by social actors, of specialized and scientific knowledge, the calculation and use of information systems and the implementation of administrative procedures and protocols. It claims that all knowledge can be expressed as a defined system. These specialized knowledge systems are applied in the context of impersonal relationships and are aimed at working towards gaining greater control over the world. The terms 'rationality' and 'rationalization' are used interchangeably by Weber (1968) to signify a characteristic of action. The term 'rationalization' is generally referred to as a process of making action, services or products more rational.

The reasons for rationalization are to fulfil the need for centralization, to create economies of scale and to produce evidence for claims of quality and efficiency (McKinlay and Arches, 1985). Rationalization serves the function of controlling the work force through producing habits of predictability, dependability, standardization and internalization of the organization's goals.

Weber (1968), however, distiguishes between two 'ideal types' of rationality: 'formal' or zweckrational rationality which is described by Simon (1957) as 'a matter of fact', and 'substantive' or wertrational rationality described by Simon (1957) as 'a matter of value'.

FORMAL RATIONALITY

Formal rationality is characterized by calculated and purposeful action chosen specifically to obtain ends; it refers primarily to the calculability of means and procedures (Fox, 1991). In its purest form it is impersonal and aims to calculate the most precise and efficient means for the resolution of problems by ordering them under abstract rules and regulations and clearly stipulated procedures (Kalberg, 1980). Kalberg (1980) argues that within formal-rational systems decisions are arrived at 'without regard to persons', arbitrariness is rejected, decision-making is strictly opposed to any reference to the personal qualities of the individuals concerned. As Weber (1968) argues:

> ... where formal rationality is maximized, its participants do not look towards the persons of each other but only toward the commodity; there are no obligations of brotherliness or reference, and none of those spontaneous human relations that are sustained by personal unions.
>
> (Weber, 1968: 636)

For example, a skill-mix review which linked activities undertaken in the home with the particular skills of the practitioner is an example of a formal-rational approach to care as it controls the workforce through applying 'scientific principles' to delegation and allocation of work. By use of the example of caseload discharge criteria, Timmins (1996) claims in her community study that she found little evidence of 'standardization' between community nurses as to when to discharge patients from their caseloads. She described 'highly predictable' post-operative surgical patients and 'less predictable long term chronic sick' patients. Through greater rationalization (for example, by using clearer and more specific discharge criteria) the consumer can receive or be denied those goods and services that officials of the organization (community nurses) are guided to produce or deny (Freidson, 1990).

By applying given discharge criteria, community nurses would be controlled by the organization which effectively reduces their autonomy and does not allow them to use their personal knowledge of their patients and their needs. As Ritzer (1994) argues, formal rationality is institutionalized in large-scale bureaucracies where workers' actions are determined by the rules and regulations of the organization rather than by their own intellectual and evaluative processes. Brubaker (1984) explains that in 'formal' rationality work is determined not only by a deliberate and impersonal quantitative calculation based on the application of standards and procedures but also the administrative separation of official and professional activites from the personal and private affairs of individuals. Therefore, decisions that are reached are free from the 'multifarious fetters of tradition and the capricious influence of feelings'. As Hillier (1987) has succinctly argued:

Officials are not self-interested. Their conduct is governed by specific rules which restrict them to certain areas of competence, and the application of laws and rules is therefore free from irrational discrimination or ignorance. The most appropriate form of administration is the bureaucracy, the impersonal power of officialdom.

(Hillier, 1987: 206)

In summary, it is claimed that formal rationality will increase in society to the extent that technically possible calculations of efficiency and cost-effectiveness will be universally applied irrespective of their effects on the needs of individuals or to the extent that they conflict with substantive rationality or the intensely personal and human values that traditionally distinguish health care (Kalberg, 1980).

SUBSTANTIVE RATIONALITY

Formal rationality is therefore opposed to the more traditional, affective, emotional and metaphysical forms of knowledge such as may be found in kinship groups such as families and close-knit communities. These qualities are described by Weber (1968), as 'substantive' rationality. Substantitive rationality is concerned with the espousal of broad human values such as social justice; ends and outcomes are seen as paramount rather than calculating the cost of achieving them. Kalberg (1980) states that values such as trust, compassion and mutual assistance constitute substantive rationality. In health care values such as altruism, professional autonomy, trust and the more recent espoused value of 'client-centredness' would constitute substantive rationalities (Ritzer and Walczak, 1988; Baggott, 1998) as they form overarching values to which actions and roles are normally subordinated.

McIntosh (1996: 319) provides examples of community nurses' substantive approach: that of using autonomy and 'regard to persons'. She describes a novice nurse as struggling with the need to be 'adaptable', as 'acting with a totally different persona' with different families, as 'carefully negotiating' her role in the home, as 'knowing very precisely' how to strike the balance between the conflicting roles of being a guest and nurse in different situations and as developing a 'repertoire of responses to use in the changing contexts of different homes'.

In spite of these examples, Weber (1968) concluded that since science and technology formed so much of modern life, formal rationalism would tend to overwhelm substantive rationalism and will come to dominate society. This would lead to an increase in secularization and a consequent decrease in affection, tradition and metaphysical systems of belief. Blau and Scott (1963) argue that organizational behaviour dictates that all decisions will become based on 'factual' rather than 'value' premises. Managers will confine their duties to selecting the most efficient means to achieve the organization's ends. Bureaucracy, seen by Weber (1968) as the epitome of rationalization, would dictate that choosing alternative means of providing a service or using specialized equipment or introducing innovation or acting autonomously (all espoused values of community nurses) is restricted by procedural regulations such as contracts and protocols.

Coles (1996) summarized that the struggle to preserve basic human values and promote social and humane aspects of life in a health care system that appears to be devoid of compassion leaves nursing effectively trapped between the two competing paradigms. Further evidence of this comes from Kirk and Glendinning (1998) who argue that community nurses are reported to feel that their autonomy, priorities and practice are determined by the requirements of the service purchasers. This produces the reality that they remain task oriented 'and give priority to the instrumental rather than the affective dimensions of care' (Kirk and Glendinning, 1998: 376).

As Weber (1968) has argued:

> Bureaucracy develops the more perfectly, the more it is 'dehumanized', the more completely it succeeds in eliminating from official business love, hatred, and all purely personal . . . and emotional elements which escape calculation.
>
> (Weber 1968: 975)

Brubaker (1984) has also argued that there is perpetual tension and often deep hostility between the formal rationality of bureacratic systems and the substantive rationality of fraternal and caritive values. Therefore to apply a formal-rational, calculating approach within the traditional informal environment of the home clearly affects the nurse–client relationship. A point the Audit Commission (1999) has noted:

> Trusts and commissioners should recognise that, with pressure to increase efficiency and the rise in technical, as opposed to personal, nursing care, there is a danger that some of the things that patients say they value most highly will be lost.
>
> (Audit Commission, 1999: 54)

Theorizing community nursing

Kelly *et al.* (1998: 165) propose that community nursing is in a dichotomous position. These authors claim that 'the day-to-day culture imposed by medicine and management promotes reductionist approaches while professional and educational pressures point to virtually opposite philosophies and values in relation to health and holism'. This chapter argues that a third element should be constructed and applied to any theory development; that of the context of care (Figure 7.1).

The Audit Commission (1999) claims that determining what constitutes 'good care' is seldom clear-cut and there are few outcome measures that can gauge standards of care. Furthermore:

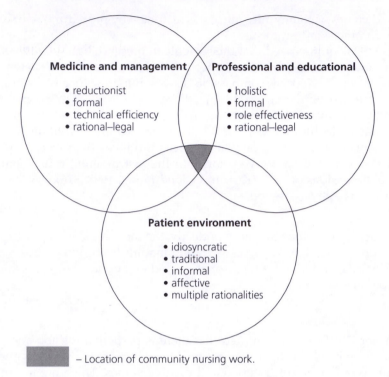

– Location of community nursing work.

Figure 7.1 Conceptual influences on community nursing

... the apparent invisibility of much [district] nursing practice means
that it is often understood in only the broadest, and most simplistic, of
terms. Its public stereotyping as an unhurried, low-tech, backwater service – a service that time forgot – is both inaccurate and undeserved.

(Audit Commission, 1999: 3)

Luker and Kenrick (1992) contend that the community base of nurses
means that their practice is often largely invisible and isolated, they can be
'out of sight and out of mind' (Audit Commission, 1999) and that, as they
rarely have the opportunity for systematic peer review, may develop idiosyncratic practices. Ong (1991) claims that the case of district nursing is particularly interesting as the location of the majority of care is carried out in the
patient's home which profoundly influences the balance between being a professional and being a guest.

When these informal and qualitative aspects of social relationships and the
non-professional and non-technical aspects of caring in the home are considered it becomes much more difficult to define the purposes of the community
nursing service and the core activities of the nurses themselves (Timmins, 1996).

It appears tempting but too simplistic to argue that community nursing is
simply the relocation of hospital nursing into the home and that the skills of
the community nurse are analogous to the skills of the hospital nurse.

McIntosh (1985) argues that the problems community nurses have in defending their specialized role arises from deep-rooted ignorance about their work. She claims there is a perception that hospital is where the 'difficult or real' nursing is done, that inpatient care is more complex and that patients are discharged when their nursing needs are thought to be reduced to a minimum. McIntosh (1985) goes on to argue that with regard to the elderly and chronically ill community nurses have a far more complex task than their hospital counterparts and that the community nurse's teaching, communication and organizing role is 'persistently denied' in favour of the image as a provider of basic nursing care. There is nothing to indicate that the findings from hospital-based studies relating to practice are transferable to community locations (Luker and Kenrick, 1992).

Furthermore there can be no equivalence between the formal, bureaucratic hospital environment and the informal social-cultural conditions in patients' own homes. In hospital, the ways in which the nurse–patient relationship is structured are related to the institutional definitions of the roles of both parties (McGilloway, 1976). In the home no such institutional definitions exist. These are not just environmental differences but include aspects of power, authority and decision-making prerogatives in the implementation of care and treatments and in the social dynamics governing the type and quality of the nurse–patient relationship. As Nettleton and Burrows (1994) have argued:

> The prime object of medical care located within the hospital was a diseased anatomy, the central object of health care located in the community is a 'whole person'. Moreover, the whole person has a voice, a view and a valid perspective which is increasingly regarded as a crucial dimension of effective health care.
>
> (Nettleton and Burrows 1994: 94)

Unlike hospital nurses, the community nurse does not have back-up services or staff to call on to provide immediate support or consultation (Coombs, 1984). Griffiths and Luker (1997) argue that the confidence required to practice alone and take decisions in isolation in the community should not be underestimated for a nurse used to working in the protected environment of the hospital. In longer term relationships in the home, particularly where chronic illness is concerned, the dimensions and dynamics of that relationship, both with patients and carers, alter significantly. This, as Hennessy and Swain (1997) state, is principally because nurses who work in people's own homes have come to respect and recognize the home as the domain of patients and their families.

The influence of the 'home' environment

In contrast to the hospital environment, Nettleton and Burrows (1994) claim that the community or home setting can be viewed conceptually as post-

Fordist which is distinguished by pluralism, decentralization and an orientation to the consumer. In other words it is informal or irrational and subject to mutiple 'value spheres' (Hillier, 1987). Twigg (1999) argues that the home can be conceptualized as a place of privacy, security, comfort and ease and as a site of personal expression:

> ... home is itself structured in terms of privacy and intimacy, with certain areas remaining relatively hidden from strangers and associated more intensely with personal life.
>
> (Twigg 1999: 383)

Unlike the hospital environment, it becomes the embodiment of identity and therefore limits the degree to which a person can become depersonalized. The social ethics of privacy and security give patients and clients the 'power to exclude' and this power conveys an element of control and hence makes it possible to resist the dominace of careworkers. It is therefore in some sense antibureaucratic. Many times during a working day community nurses have to cross into this private world and make continual adjustments to the idiosyncratic territories that are 'complex, cultural constructs embodying both material and ideological aspects' (Twigg 1999: 385). Furthermore, in the spacial ordering within the home, community nurses frequently gain entry to the most private, intimate and hidden areas: the bedroom, bathroom and toilet (Twigg, 1999) and carry out intimate or technical procedures that would normally be confined to the bureaucratic conditions of the doctor's surgery, outpatient clinic or ward treatment room.

Within the hospital environment McGilloway (1976) has detailed the difficulties:

> The practitioner deals with people in situations which involve intimacies, that is, in contexts which are often considered 'private' to the patient himself. To touch, manipulate and expose the body of another are carefully regulated activities in most societies . . . It is essential, but remains a privilege, for the practitioner to have access to the body of another. Indeed some of her contacts . . . would not be permitted to any other person by most normal individuals, even sexual partners.
>
> (McGilloway, 1976:)

Within the covert, non-institutional context of the home, where people live their daily lives and rest, work, or entertain, the conflict in crossing social taboos is significantly heightened. Community nurses would recognize the significant cultural dissonance of this and have empathy because of their own shared values of their own homes (Twigg, 1999). They would acknowledge their intrusion into the private domain of the patient (Hennessy and Swain, 1997) and see that the actions of professional dominance are nullified as the patient or carer has the ultimate sanction of allowing or refusing their admittance. Community nurses need to maintain a perspective of respect for the person's dominance in their own homes and should reserve their own personal judgements about, for example, cleanliness, tidyness and clinical suitability. They have to 'act as a strong antidote to an exclusive bio-medical and evidence-based clinical effective model' (Hennessy and Swain, 1997: 13). They are, in effect, deprofessionalized as they do not fully control the care environment and their expert knowledgeable actions and professional standards can be ignored, compromised or undone by patients in their absence.

It is this ingredient of a traditional and irrational environment and the necessity for community nurses to exist within it that may indicate reasons for the non-confrontational, courtesy-based 'etiquette' which develops within some branches of community nursing and can become a barrier to achieving clinical effectiveness (Griffiths and Luker, 1997).

The home is therefore anti-bureaucratic as rational rules cannot be wholly applied and there can be no or little separation of the official activities of the community nurse from the private affairs of the patient as Hillier (1987) proposed earlier. Providing health care in the home therefore has to be idiosyncratic because of the 'sheer diversity to be found in people's home environments, lifestyles, family and neighbourhood support systems' (Bryans and McIntosh, 1996: 25). Protocols and procedures cannot be followed rigidly as many of the problems encountered by community nurses are of an uncertain and ill-structured nature. Patients cannot be seen merely as biological systems; they are set within their families and communities and within the context of their own homes with all the attendant social, personal and emotional needs, wants and activities. They form social relationships and friendships with those with whom they come into contact (Davy, 1998). This is much more likely when any kind of helping relationship is regular and ongoing.

The views of patients

Patients and clients have been found not to distinguish between the physical and social-psychological aspects of their illness. They consider that their illness pervades other aspects of their lives and that it is the remit of community nurses to deal with the totality of their need (Ong, 1991). Despite their power to exclude carers, patients also realize that their power is weakened since they are in a dependent relationship with their care providers. They are often vulnerable through their lack of knowledge, lack of skills and debilitated physical and emotional state. Vulnerablility and dependence are stigmatized states not usually expected in the home environment which epitomizes independence, self-sufficiency and individuality and patients frequently employ social techniques to gain knowledge about, understanding of and hence acceptability with their care providers. These 'mutual self-disclosures' are aimed at attaining equality in the relationship (Hunt, 1991).

Small, qualitative studies have uncovered some of these social processes. Ong (1991) found that patients empathized with the problems community nurses encountered in their work as their 'understanding' engendered a positive response from the practitioner. Coombs (1984) noted that, by its nature, primary nursing develops exclusivity in the nurse–patient relationship and in the community this is often accentuated where the nurse frequently became 'a window through which the patient views the outside world' (Coombs, 1984: 161).

The Audit Commission (1999) drew attention to this feature:

> The humanity of the [district] nursing service is fundamentally important to patients. Patients describe the value that they place on their relationships with the nurses. Liking and trusting someone on whom you are dependent and establishing a one-to-one relationship *which extends beyond the nurse's professional role* are regarded as central to the quality of their care.
>
> (Audit Commission, 1999: 53; para 109 [emphasis added])

It may now be possible to add a third dimension to the 'dichotomous' position of Kelly *et al.* (1998), the influence of the patients' environment, and this is shown in Figure 7.1. Once inside patients' environment of the home, the community nurse is in a further equivocal position in adopting certain role formats. Hunt (1991) described four role formats used by community nurses specializing in symptom control for terminally ill cancer patients: bureaucratic, bio-medical, social therapy and friendly informal. Table 7.1 aims to develop the 'different approach' needed in community nursing by incorporating aspects from the 'bureaucratic' and 'friendly informal' formats, together with concepts from Twigg (1989), Bauman (1990) and McGilloway (1976). The different approach can be seen as one of irrationality, that is, non-bureaucratic relations based on affectivity and drawing on a personal/social model of human relations. The relationship may be based on informal, personal knowledge. Here, the moral norm of reciprocity and the relevance and importance of reciprocal relations may engage the social actors and will now be considered.

The concept of reciprocity

Morse (1991) has argued that generally the relationship between the nurse and the patient is the result of 'covert interactive negotiations' between two persons. In a similar way to Hunt (1991) above, she has classified relationships within four levels: clinical, therapeutic, connected and over-involved. These levels intensify over six continua, including time-span, interaction type and patient need, and patient trust; in the home these aspects can be accentuated producing a more 'connected' relationship. It has been argued throughout this chapter that in the community, the context of care and of the nurse–patient, nurse–carer relationship is in the informal, social, affective, irrational and non-technical environment of the home; an environment which is more covert than the hospital and in which the professional practitioner cannot wholly control and, by implication, an environment in which the achievement of aims is dependent on some form of negotiation and exchange.

Table 7.1 The dichotomous position of community nurses in the home – role formats*

Formal, bureaucratic, professional role	Informal, home, 'beyond' professional role
Rational–technical authority	Socio-cultural
Universalistic	Particularistic
Affectively neutral	Affectivity
Procedural rules of care	Individualized care
Assessment of need separated from personal characteristics	Personal, ascriptive assessment of needs
Formal knowledge base (trained, technical)	Knowledge base rooted in daily, private experience
Specific care related to needs	Diffuse care
Reciprocity – equivalent exchange	Reciprocity – gift

Derived from McGilloway (1976), Twigg (1989), Bauman (1990) and Hunt (1991)

The concept of social exchange or reciprocity is fundamental to civilization and is a basic human ritual in all cultures and religions. Neufeld and Harrison (1995) define reciprocity as the bi-directional exchange of valued resources between individuals. At its simplest, the concept of reciprocity implies that there is a general expectation to make some return or exchange for goods, services or favours received as part of an ongoing and two-way process (Finch and Mason, 1993). It can be summed up in idioms such as 'one good deed deserves another' and 'a debt of gratitude'.

Gouldner (1960), in his seminal work on reciprocity, claims that social equilibrium, cohesion and stability could not exist without the 'reciprocity of service and return of service'. As a basis for his argument he cites the philosopher Cicero as saying 'there is no duty more indispenable than that of returning a kindness', yet he states that few concepts in sociology remain more obscure and ambiguous.

Wentowski (1981) claimed that the strength of reciprocity depends on several relationship characteristics, including its nature, duration and function which reflect Morse's (1991) continua. Familial relationships of long duration and emotional closeness develop reciprocity of the most general and non-specific type characterized by high levels of general commitment and enduring obligations (Antonucci and Jackson, 1989). Non-familial relations, which tend to have shorter duration, are characterized by limited feelings of reciprocity in response to a specific act of service, kindness or support. Because of the nature of community nursing it is possible that nurses' work can generate reciprocity between both ends of this scale.

Cheal (1987) implies that gifts are a symbol or measure of the relationship between the giver and the recipient and are a means through which individuals communicate the values which they assign to significant others. If given ritually they can signify close involvement and connectedness to another or be evidence of an ongoing relationship but any instance of gift-giving can be full of social significance and can have symbolic as well as material value and meaning. Maus (1954) underlines the substantive values in gift-giving. He claimed that 'to give something is to give part of oneself . . . a part of one's nature and substance, while to receive something is to receive a part of some-one's spiritual essence' (p. 10).

Reciprocity, however, is also encumbered with moral beliefs and cultural obligations. Spiker (1984) argued that it is now a 'prescribed' practice imply-ing that over time it has been tried, repeated, found to be good and useful and hence accepted as a moral imperative. It thus becomes internalized as 'nor-mative' behaviour. Henley and Schott (1999) claim that in some cultures it is common to show gratitude by giving presents or money and for this to be refused can create offence. Uehara (1995) discusses evidence that people feel obligated to return benefits they receive from others and therefore reciprocity is a fundamental principle of social organization and functional theory. Blau (1967) claims that an individual who supplies rewarding services to another obligates him and to discharge that obligation the second must furnish bene-fits to the first in turn. As Gouldner (1960) states:

> We owe others certain things because of what they have previously done for us, because of the history of previous interaction we have had with them. It is this kind of obligation which is entailed by the general-ized norm of reciprocity.
>
> (Gouldner, 1960: 171)

Anthropologists believe that gifts originated as a traditional way to con-duct trade within primitive societies (Ahuja, 1997); however, in modern 'rational' economies the use of money has removed the need for gifts in sys-tems of exchange. This implies that gift-giving is even more crucial to main-tain stable human relationships where 'kindness' or a 'service' can not be costed. Exchange theory implies that reciprocal gifts should be roughly of the same value – the principle of fairness – and that people should not overben-efit or underbenefit from the practice.

Uehara (1995) claims that there are immediate problems in situations in which there are power differences between the actors involved in the exchange and where equivalent exchange cannot be made. In these situations recipients become indebted to givers and thus dependent on them. Gouldner (1960) ends his seminal text by asserting that 'Clearly the moral norm of reciprocity cannot apply in relations with children, old people, or with those who are . . . physically handicapped' (p. 583), yet this will not prevent people feeling indebted to certain types of service provision. Spiker (1984) points out that when people are unable to reciprocate they are bound to feel grateful for what they have received which puts them at a disadvantage to the giver as gratitude is difficult to redeem; the esteem they feel towards the giver is a form of homage which enhances the giver's status and diminishes their own. Spiker (1984) summarizes:

> A person who receives something has a duty to reciprocate. If he fails to do so, an obligation is outstanding – which, by definition, implies a relative loss of status. Someone who is absolutely dependent on others, and unable to contribute anything in return, has in consequence a very low status.
>
> (Spiker, 1984: 99)

Blau (1967) also claims that:

> A person who fails to reciprocate favours is accused of ingratitude. This very accusation indicates that reciprocation is expected and it serves as a social sanction that discourages individuals from forgetting their obligations to associates. Generally, people are grateful for favours and repay their social debts, and both their gratitude and their repayment are social rewards for the associate who has done them favours.
>
> (Blau, 1967: 16)

The relationship between carer and cared-for can become a relation of dominance and disempowerment for the cared-for where they lose status and become 'the lesser, asking party' (de Swann, 1990). Greenberg (1980) argues that feelings of indebtedness are noxious and are actively avoided by individuals. In some cultures, the terms *please* and *thank you* are not used towards people who are simply doing the jobs for which they are paid (Bowler, 1993).

Fox (1993) claims that 'a gift is threatening because it establishes an inequality, a difference, an imbalance of power' (p. 95). However, to turn this point around, the gift may be seen as an attempt to return the balance of power to equilibrium, to reduce the inequality and to regain status and self-esteem. The notion that reciprocity can be a means or strategy of gaining lost self-esteem and dependency or of enhancing status and re-asserting control over one's environment appears not to have been highlighted in the nursing literature and it contrasts with the analyses of some writers, for example Chalmers (1992) and Morse (1991).

In community nursing, dependency of patients on the service is commonplace but this dependency can be acceptable since contributions have already been made through the payment of taxes or insurance and previous work status. Spiker (1984) discussed evidence that most people saw social services as residual systems to be used legitimately when individuals were unable to help themselves. The payment of taxes and insurance may signify payment for services but this is on a 'contract-by-proxy' basis and is undertaken perhaps many years before the actual exchange of service. As discussed earlier, providing community nursing care in the home, particularly for chronic conditions, is unlike using or employing any other type of domiciliary service since, for example, the duration of contact is unknown; the work, which involves physical, social and emotional aspects, is diffuse and may fluctuate in intensity; although the work may be clinical it is also personal, therapeutic and often private and intimate and frequently crosses social taboos as it is work done *to* as well as *for* the recipient. The often long-term nature of the relationship, that it occurs in the home and that it involves a caring, supportive and personal dimension influences its location on the binary opposition continuum from formal, professional-based relations to informal 'friendship' and 'kinship' relations.

Reciprocity in community nursing

Chalmers (1992) refers to 'exchange theory' within the patterns of interactions between health visitors and their clients. Such exchange can be evidenced in the phrase 'The health visitor 'gives' her service and, in exchange, the client is expected to 'give back' information and interest' (p. 1323). Although this is a type of exchange within reciprocity theory, this section concentrates specifically on the giving of gifts.

It has been pointed out earlier that the receiving of gifts which may influence the provision of care is contrary to nurses' code of professional conduct (UKCC, 1992). Studies which examined this particular dimension of the nurse–patient relationship could be not be found. However, within studies which focused on the nurse–patient relationship, particularly in the community, data can be uncovered that shows that this covert practice is enacted and in certain circumstances may be commonplace. Furthermore, social desirability and legal adherence may prohibit respondents (either patients or nurses) from admitting in any detail to the practice, and researchers from drawing attention to the phenomenon in their publications. If the notion of reciprocity is important to the functioning of social relations it deserves more attention in the literature. Since examining reciprocity was seldom the main focus of the studies, where necessary, verbatim accounts are used here to identify its existence.

Cain (1995), in his analysis of community nurse–client relations, discusses the relevance of a 'friendship' relation model in community nursing. He explains that a community nurse will meet a patient and/or carer and there may be a strong mutual liking and enjoyment of each other's company. This may lead to mutual disclosure of private matters, a concern for the welfare of one another and enquiry about loved ones and other personal aspects of life. However, Cain (1995) argues that mutual liking runs counter to the requirements of professional impartiality; it is not a requirement of care. In developing the notion of friendship, he suggests that a model might involve a 'professional friendship' where the professional could be a friend 'to' the client rather than a friend 'of' the client. He ends by posing some questions that are relevant to this discussion of reciprocity:

Should the community nurse accept gifts? Should she agree to being godmother to a client's offspring? How much self-disclosure is appropriate? In other words, at what point does 'the role of a friend' run up against other requirements of the professional role? Here, without doubt is a grey area in which community nurses may have to make ethically difficult decisions.

(Cain, 1995: 33)

Attention has already been drawn to the assertion by the Audit Commission (1999) that patients particularly valued their relationship with nurses when it extended 'beyond the professional', although what was meant by this was not defined. In her small, qualitative study Davy (1998) showed that most respondents felt that community nurses were friends to them and felt a particular warmth when the nurse had performed a caring behaviour 'over and above what was expected of them'. She later described this as nurses providing 'extras' or 'going the extra mile'. 'Going the extra mile' was a term Morse (1991) used to describe the 'connected' level relationship of a home care nurse which had grown 'beyond a clinical and therapeutic relationship' and which developed either through extreme need or through a long-term relationship.

Poole and Rowat (1994) discussed perceptions of a caring home care nurse. They noted that elderly clients in particular suffered from social isolation and reported issues of lack of social contact and the need for encouragement from their nurses. The issue of a right to self-determination was important for them and was often achieved through reciprocity – their need and power to give back something to their nurses:

Reciprocity issues focused on *the client's need to give something in return for the services provided*. Examples of reciprocity ranged from clients enquiring about the nurses' holidays to the offering of small gifts or food.

(Poole and Rowat, 1994: 426 [emphasis added])

Here, reciprocity, expressed as a social need, could be claimed to be a therapeutic element within the relationship and to refuse a gift would deny clients their right to self-determination in their own homes. Trojan and Young (1993) discuss the same theme. They examined the process of how home care nurses developed a trusting relationship and claim that:

Trusting, caring relationships is the core category which encompasses the trust which is developed, as well as the nursing care that is provided. Nurses provide care to their clients, helping them to live independently in their own homes and *clients reciprocate in their own ways*.

(Trojan and Young, 1993: 1904 [emphasis added[)

Using grounded theory methods, Trojan and Young (1993) identified the phase of 'initial trusting', a theme of which was 'accepting'. Here:

Nurses accepted the clients' homes, cultures, lifestyles, decisions, refusal of services and offers of coffee. If a nurse could not accept the clients and their values, the development of a trusting nurse–patient relationship was impeded.

(Trojan and Young, 1993: 1905)

Thorne and Robinson (1988) discussed strategies which some chronically ill patients used to develop intimate and collegial relationships with carefully selected health care professionals:

The final strategy by which informants used their newly acquired competence to foster trust involved efforts to reduce the status differential between themselves and their health care professionals. The informants described gift-giving, inquiring about the professional's health and family life, joking, expressing concern for the professional's working conditions . . .

(Thorne and Robinson, 1988: 786)

This strategy was used by patients who were chronically ill as a means of collaboration and co-operation; an attempt to equalize the relationship with care providers. Thorne and Robinson (1988), however, claimed that health professionals were resistant to incorporate reciprocity into their relationships as the social distance between patients and providers served as a mechanism to preserve their authority. Morse (1991) suggested a different tack. She claimed there was a hidden agenda in gift-giving and that 'many of the strategies used by patients in coercive or manipulative relationships to ensure nursing care, [were] the giving of gifts or bribes . . . ' (p. 462).

Hunt (1991) discusses the tensions community nurses have in trying to balance their professional, authoritarian role whilst in the informal setting of the home:

Because the nurses were working in patients' homes, they seemed to be trying to achieve a balance between the 'informality' inherent in the context, such as being given cups of tea, coping with the presence of pets and children, and presenting themselves authoritatively.

(Hunt, 1991: 936)

Hunt (1991) claims that features of 'being friendly' can be displayed through presentational skills, such as smiling, tone of voice and use of social talk, but these are superficial compared to those attributed to 'friendship'. Friendships are characterized by reciprocity, interdependence and equity 'with the exchange of personal and intimate information and feel-ings'. Although there is evidence of self-disclosure in the literature, Hunt (1991) argues that the claim made by professionals to becoming friends with patients is problematic and needs questioning since professional–client situations do not fulfil the requirements of friendships. The UKCC (1999) is circumspect in its advice. It claims that the nurse–client relation-ship is 'not established to build personal or social contacts for practitioners' and recognizes that nurses and health visitors 'may, on occasions, develop strong feelings for a particular client or family' but adds that 'these feelings in themselves are neither abnormal or wrong' (p. 5).

Although not a study involving community nurses, Clarke and Wheeler (1992) investigated the meaning of care in a small study of staff nurses in a British hospital. The nurses emphasized the humanistic experiences of care in phrases such as 'the giving of self, valuing people, respect, trust and loving concern'. They claimed that the giving of self was very prominent in all the informants' responses but more important was the understanding that the nurse would 'not only give of herself but gain something from the process by so doing'. Furthermore:

> The nurses' giving of themselves . . . was recognized as fundamental to caring. This involved physical, psychological and emotional giving, with the voluntary sharing of themselves through disclosing personal information. Such a process develops friendship with the patients as people and the evolution of mutual trust.
>
> (Clarke and Wheeler, 1992: 1287)

Timmins (1996) uncovers the dilemmas of preserving social distance in her study of discharge processes within community nursing. She admits that com-munity nursing emerged as an intensely human experience in which strong emotional attachments could develop between members of the nursing team and their patients and carers. Some staff felt tension in trying to negotiate a relationship that did not result in attachment or obligation. Although gift-giving was not openly discussed, it is implied when one district nurse is quoted as saying 'Its like accepting things from a rep [company representa-tive], you know that sort of, "Well you've had my meal you can't say no."'

However, another staff member in the study considered that 'strong attach-ments between her and her team members and patients gave a richness of care'. Timmins (1996) explains that interactions may take place on the basis of rewards and that in this context 'rewards' may be an increasingly rich friend-ship based on increasing self-disclosure and later adds 'a number of nurses described forms of attachment involving, for example, the sharing of meals with patients . . . ' She argued that these exchanges 'are rather more than an exchange of particular goods but part of a moral transaction'. Food as a gift is in a special category. Lupton (1996) describes it as the ultimate gift since it is both symbolically and physiologically consumed and nourishes both the body and the psyche.

Morse (1991), however, criticized what she described as 'over-involved relationships' where they develop 'beyond a professional relationship' and are characterized by loss of objectivity which overrides nurses' commitment to the treatment regime and their responsibility to other patients and where they come to be treated as members of their patients' families.

Classifying reciprocal acts

Gouldner (1960) described the concept of reciprocity as 'ambiguous'. Although Morse's (1991) project began as a study of gift-giving as a response to care in the patient–nurse relationship, she claimed that during the data analysis 'it became clear that the gift was merely a symbol of the type of relationship developed'. The study therefore developed to analyse and classify nurse–patient relationships.

The evidence from this chapter seems to point to three main facets of reciprocity which have differing origins and can be conceptualized differently.

RECIPROCITY AS A LEGITIMATE EXPRESSION OF GRATITUDE

A gift in this situation would be symbolic of the end of the care episode, the treatment regimen and the therapeutic relationship. This can be seen as normative behaviour on the hospital ward where chocolates, flowers or a financial contribution to ward funds are given as a public expression of thanks. No coercive influence would be measured and the gesture would not be seen as influencing future care. Acceptance of the neutrality of the gift is further assured since its focus is often not to an individual but diffused across the nursing and medical teams.

In the community, this process is less open but may be through a letter to a manager or the delivery of a gift directly to the health centre. Frequently gifts symbolising the end of care are given directly to the visiting nurses while still in the home. In this context, the giving and receiving of gifts is covert.

RECIPROCITY AS A STRATEGY TO GAIN FAVOURS

Here, gift-giving may be part of a hierarchy of strategies employed to influence the type, range and intensity of care. This may begin with examples of personal disclosure as discussed earlier and escalate to covert gift-giving to individual staff during an episode of care. The influential nature of the action is open to interpretation and to separate expressions of gratitude from actions of influence may be difficult to achieve.

The effectiveness of this strategy is also debateable as Morse (1991) claimed that this practice actually increased nurse–patient distance. It is this type of reciprocity that the UKCC (1992) cautions against because of its aim to 'obtain preferential consideration'.

RECIPROCITY AS A MEANS TO REGAIN STATUS

This would appear to be a genuine, but thus far, neglected role of gift-giving. Reciprocity may be seen as a benign social strategy that patients use to achieve or regain a balance in status with their caregivers. It is a strategy of exerting self-determination and a means to regain independence and a degree of equality and control within the partnership of care. It may be a key part of patients' rehabilitative and recovery processes similar in importance to walking post-operatively or getting dressed in their own clothes. This strategy is more likely to occur in the home environment where self-care is encouraged and the patient may be used to being in control. The hospital ward can disempower and strip away all personal and individual characteristics. In the home, which is the seat of individual expression and personal authority, gift-giving may be a simple but profound act of self-expression where the recipient may actually be an insignificant part of the equation.

Conclusion

This chapter has attempted to outline the position of the community nurse working in the environment of patients' homes. Community nurses are subjected to opposing formal and informal forces which can, on the one hand, constrain and delimit their role through the focus on technical and task data, but on the other, encourage close, personal and rewarding relationships with patients and carers though these may not be valued by current medical and management models.

A bureaucratic, formal, universalistic and normative approach protects the nurse against developing a close personal relationship with the patient as personal friendship can be seen as running counter to the ideology of professional behaviour (McGilloway 1976). However:

> The impetus for promoting 'informality' and 'friendliness' in nurse–patient relationships seems motivated by desires to break down traditional, authoritarian, professional-client barriers, thus creating more equitable encounters and 'partnerships'.
>
> (Hunt, 1991)

In situations of long-term care and chronic illness, where patients, clients and their carers may feel they wish to reciprocate because they are genuinely grateful for the service received or in order not to feel so dependent or indebted to their professional carers, or because they wish to reinstate their self-esteem, to offer a gift (and have their gift accepted) may cause them satisfaction and pleasure. To refuse a gift may prevent the development of the therapeutic relationship and create a barrier between the nurse and the patient.

Can gift-giving and receiving be interpreted as 'seeking to exert influence to obtain preferential consideration?' (UKCC, 1992). If the answer to this question is 'No' then the code of professional conduct allows the giving and receiving of gifts from patients and clients since the planning of health care should always be given on the basis of need. Reciprocity has been shown to be an important aspect of all social relations, not just between friends as is suggested in some of the literature examined, and is seen as a significant way of expressing gratitude and showing feelings.

The research available has not considered this particular aspect of community nursing. Most studies have discovered data from professional health practitioners rather than from patients and careful reading of these has uncovered some indication of the practice of gift giving and receiving. Further research could examine the views of patients and carers: what motivates them to reciprocate when the end of the care is not in sight? Is the giving of gifts therapeutic for them? To what extent do they view gift-giving as 'bribery' or an attempt to gain special favours? Does gift-giving occur in all of Morse's (1991) and Hunt's (1991) categories? Does gift-receiving foretell the end of being 'professional'?

These are potentially interesting and valuable areas of research which could further develop the theory of nurse-client relations, particularly in the less formal and client-controlled environment of the home.

References

Ahuja, A. (1997) The ritual of giving. The Times. 15 December; 10.

Antonucci, T. and Jackson, J. (1989) Successful ageing and life course reciprocity. In: Warnes. A. (ed.) *Human ageing and later life*. London: Edward Arnold; 83–95.

Audit Commission. (1992) *Homeward bound – a new course for community health*. London: Audit Commission.

Audit Commission. (1999) *First assessment: a review of district nursing services in England and Wales*. London: Audit Commission.

Bauman, Z. (1990) *Thinking sociologically*. Oxford: Blackwell.

Blau, P. (1967) *Exchange and power in social life*. New York: John Wiley & Sons.

Blau, P. and Scott, W. (1963) *Formal organizations – a comparative approach*. London: Routledge & Kegan Paul.

Bowler, I. (1993) Stereotypes of women of Asian descent in midwifery: some evidence. *Midwifery*, 9: 7–16.

Brubaker, R. (1984) *The limits of rationality. An essay on the social and moral thought of Max Weber*. London: George Allen & Unwin.

Bryans, A. and McIntosh, J. (1996) Decision making in community nursing: an analysis of the stages of decision making as they relate to community nursing assessment practice. *Journal of Advanced Nursing*, 24: 24–30.

Burley, S., Mitchell, E. and Melling K. *et al.* (1997) *Contemporary community nursing*. London: Arnold.

Cain, P. (1995) Community nurse–client relations. In: Cain, P., Hyde, V. and Howkins, E. (eds) *Community nursing – dimensions and dilemmas*. London: Arnold; 27–41.

Cain, P., Hyde, V. and Howkins, E. (eds) *Community nursing: dimensions and dilemmas*. London: Arnold.

Chalmers. K. (1992) Giving and receiving: an empirically derived theory on health visiting practice. *Journal of Advanced Nursing*, 17: 1317–25.

Cheal, D. (1987) 'Showing them that you love them': gift giving and the dialectic of intimacy. *Sociological Review*, 35: 150–69.

Clarke, J. and Wheeler, S. (1992) A view of the phenomenon of caring in nursing practice. *Journal of Advanced Nursing*, 17: 1283–90.

Coles, L. (1996) Clinical care at home. In: Gastrell, P. and Edwards, J. (eds) *Community health nursing – frameworks for practice*. London: Bailliere Tindall; 246–58.

Coombs, E. (1984) A conceptual framework for home nursing. *Journal of Advanced Nursing*, 9: 157–63.

Davy, M. (1998) Patients' views of the care given by district nurses. *Professional Nurse*, 13: 498–502.

Department of Health (DOH). (1989a) *Working for patients*. Cm 555. London: HMSO.

Department of Health (DOH). (1989b) *Caring for people*. Cm 849. London: HMSO.

Department of Health (DOH). (1997) *The new NHS – modern and dependable*. London: The Stationery Office.

Department of Health (DOH). (1998a) *Our healthier nation*. London: The Stationery Office.

Department of Health (DOH). (1998b) *Health and personal social services for England – 1998 edition*. London: The Stationery Office.

Department of Health and Social Security (DHSS). (1986) *Neighbourhood nursing: a focus for care, report of the community nursing review (the Cumberlege Report)*. London: HMSO.

de Swann, A. (1990) *The management of normality*. London: Routledge.

Finch, J. and Groves, J. (1993) *Negotiating family responsibilities*. London: Tavistock/Routledge.

Fox, N. (1991) Postmodernism, rationality and the evaluation of health care. *Sociological Review*, 39: 709–44.

Fox, N. (1993) *Postmodernism, sociology and health*. Buckingham: Open University Press.

Freidson, E. (1990) The centrality of professionalism to health care. *Jurimetrics Journal*, Summer, 431–45.

Goodman, C. (1996) District nursing and the National Health Service reforms: a case for clarification. *Journal of Nursing Management*, 4: 207–12.

Gouldner, A. (1960) The norm of reciprocity: a preliminary statement. *American Sociological Review*, 25: 161–78.

Greenberg, M. (1980) A theory of indeptedness. In: Gergen, K., Greenberg, M. and Willis, R. (eds) *Social exchange: advances in theory and research*. New York: Plenum Press; 3–26.

Griffiths, J. and Luker, K. (1997) A barrier to clinical effectiveness: the etiquette of district nursing. *Journal of Clinical Effectiveness in Nursing*, 1: 121-30.

Haste, F. and Macdonald, L. (1992) The role of the specialist in community nursing: perceptions of specialist and district nurses. *International Journal of Nursing Studies*, 29: 37–47.

Henley, A. and Schott, J. (1999) *Culture, religion and patient care in a multi-ethnic society*. London: Age Concern England.

Hennessy, D. (ed.) (1997) *Community health care development*. Basingstoke: Macmillan.

Hennessy, D. and Swain, G. (1997) Developing community health care. In: Hennessy, D. (ed.) *Community health care development*. Basingstoke: Macmillan; 3–36.

Hillier, S. (1987) Rationalism, bureacracy, and the organisation of the health services: Max Weber's contribution to understanding modern health care systems. In: Scambler, G. (ed.) *Sociological theory and medical sociology*. London: Tavistock Publications, 195–220.

Hunt, M. (1991) Being friendly and informal: reflected in nurses', terminally ill patients' and relatives' conversations in the home. *Journal of Advanced Nursing*, 16: 929–38.

Hyde, V. (1995) Community nursing: a unified discipline? In: Cain, P., Hyde, V. and Howkins, E. (eds) *Community nursing – dimensions and dilemmas*. London: Arnold; 1–26.

Kalberg, S. (1980) Weber's types of rationality. *American Journal of Sociology*, 85: 1145–79.

Kelly, A., Mabbett, G. and Thom, R. (1998) Professions and community nursing. In: Symonds, A. and Kelly, A. (eds) *The social construction of community care*. Basingstoke: Macmillan; 157–75.

Kirk, S. and Glendinning, C. (1998) Trends in community care: implications for the roles of informal carers and community nurses in the United Kingdom. *Journal of Advanced Nursing*, 28: 370–81.

Kratz, C. (1976) Some determinants of care of patients with stroke who were nursed in their own homes. *Journal of Advanced Nursing*, 1: 89–96.

Luker, K. and Kenrick, M. (1992) An exploratory study of sources of influences on the clinical decisions of community nurses. *Journal of Advanced Nursing*, 17: 457–66.

Lupton, D. (1996) *Food, the body and the self*. London: Sage Publications.

Maus, M. (1990) *The gift: the form and reason for exchange in archaic societies*. (Trans: Halls W.D.) London: Routledge.

McGilloway, F. (1976) Dependency and vulnerability in the nurse/patient situation. *Journal of Advanced Nursing*, 1: 229–36.

McIntosh, J. (1985) District nursing: a case of political marginality. In: White, R. (ed.) *Political issues in nursing: past, present and future*. Chichester: John Wiley & Sons.

McIntosh, J. (1996) The question of knowledge in district nursing. *International Journal of Nursing Studies*, 33: 316–24.

McKinlay, J. and Arches, J. (1985) Towards the proletarianisation of physicians. *International Journal of Health Services*, 16: 161–95.

Morse, J. (1991) Negotiating commitment and involvement in the nurse–patient relationship. *Journal of Advanced Nursing*, 16: 455–68.

National Health Service (NHS) Executive. (1998) *The new NHS – modern and dependable – developing primary care groups*. London: DOH.

National Health Service (NHS) Management Executive. (1993) *New world, new opportunities – nursing in primary health care*. London: DOH.

Nettleton, S. and Burrows, R. (1994) From bodies in hospitals to people in the community: a theoretical analysis of the relocation of health care. *Care in Place*, 1: 93–103.

Neufeld, A. and Harrison, M. (1995) Reciprocity and social support in caregivers' relationships: variations and consequences. *Qualitative Health Research*, 5: 348–65.

Ong, B.N. (1991) Researching needs in district nursing. *Journal of Advanced Nursing*, 17: 638–47.

Poole, G. and Rowat, K. (1994) Elderly clients' perceptions of caring of a home-care nurse. *Journal of Advanced Nursing*, 20: 422–9.

Ritzer, G. (1994) *Sociological beginings: on the origins of key ideas in sociology*. New York: McGraw-Hill.

Ritzer, G. and Walczak, D. (1988) Rationalization and the deprofessionalization of physicians. *Social Forces*, 67: 1–22.

Ross, F. and Mackenzie, A. (1996) *Nursing in primary health care: policy into practice.* London: Routledge.

Schon, D. (1983) *The reflective practitioner.* New York: Basic Books.

Simon, H. (1957) *Administrative behaviour* (second edition). New York: Macmillan.

Sines, D. (ed.) (1995) *Community health care nursing.* Oxford: Blackwell Science.

Skidmore, D. (1997) *Community care: initial training and beyond.* London: Arnold.

Spiker, P. (1984) *Stigma and social welfare.* London: Croom Helm.

Thorne, S. and Robinson, C. (1988) Reciprocal trust in health care relationships. *Journal of Advanced Nursing*, 13: 728–89.

Timmins, A. (1996) *Dilemmas of discharge: the case of district nursing.* Nottingham: Department of Nursing and Midwifery Studies, University of Nottingham.

Trojan, L. and Young, O. (1993) Developing trusting, caring relationships: home care nurses and elderly clients. *Journal of Advanced Nursing*, 18: 1903–10.

Twigg, J. (1989) Models of carers: how do social care agencies conceptualise their relationship with informal carers. *Journal of Social Policy*, 18: 53–66.

Twigg, J. (1999) The spatial ordering of care: public and private in bathing support at home. *Sociology of Health and Illness*, 21: 381–400.

Twinn, S., Roberts, B. and Andrews, S. (1996) *Community health nursing: principles for practice.* Oxford: Butterworth Heinemann.

Uehara, E. (1995) Reciprocity reconsidered: Gouldner's 'moral norm of reciprocity' and social support. *Journal of Social and Personal Relationships*, 12: 483–502.

United Kingdom Central Council (UKCC). (1992) *Code of professional conduct for the nurse, midwife and health visitor* (third edition). London: UKCC.

United Kingdom Central Council (UKCC). (1994) *The future of professional practice – the Council's standards for education and practice following registration.* London: UKCC.

United Kingdom Central Council (UKCC). (1998) *Standards for specialist education and practice: Registrar's letter 11/1998.* London: UKCC.

United Kingdom Central Council (UKCC). (1999) *Practitioner–client relationships and the prevention of abuse.* London: UKCC.

Weber, M. (1968) *Economy and society.* New Jersey: Bedminster Press.

Wentowski, G. (1981) Reciprocity and the coping strategies of older people: cultural dimensions of network building. *The Gerontologist*, 21: 6000–9.

8 Autonomous roles in the community

Rosie Walsh

Introduction

Primary care is facing a time of rapid change and the climate for innovation and development has been encouraged by the government's willingness initially to consider personal medical services pilot sites, with particular emphasis on the development of nurse-led services (Marchant *et al.*, 1997; DOH, 1997a, 1997b, 1998a). In 1999, the White Paper, *Making a Difference* (DOH, 1999c), also emphasized the need to strengthen the nursing, midwifery and health visiting contribution to healthcare with initiatives such as nurse consultant posts and extended nursing roles. Primary care groups (PCGs), established since the introduction of the White Paper, *The New NHS – Modern and Dependable* (DOH, 1997c), have been able to influence local primary care services and will be able to flex practitioners and resources once they become free-standing Trusts at levels 3 and 4 (DOH, 1997a, 1998b). First-wave trusts came into being in April 2000 (DOH, 1999a). The recent Green Paper, *Our Healthier Nation* (DOH, 1998c), and subsequent White Paper, *Saving Lives: Our Healthier Nation* (DOH, 1999d) have highlighted the need to tackle health inequalities and develop services for deprived people and to meet unmet needs. Educational courses for nurses working at an advanced level also appear to have proliferated since their introduction in the late 1980s. The current drop in the number of general practitioners (GPs), particularly working in inner city areas, has also encouraged the development of extended nursing roles (Chapple *et al.*, 1999). Recent innovations facilitating the development of such roles also include walk-in centres (DOH, 1999e), out-of-hours services (DOH, 1995) and NHS Direct (DOH, 1999f, 1999g). In light of all these factors, it appears particularly opportune to explore autonomous practice and the variety of extended roles which are developing in the community.

Defining autonomy

The concept of autonomy appears complex and difficult to define. It is perhaps more easy to describe in relation to physiological processes where autonomy characterizes a process that is independent of normal regulatory mechanisms, such as the autonomic nervous system which functions mainly independently of conscious will (Shotter, 1975; Tortora and Grabowski, 1996; Wilkinson, 1997). Personal autonomy, however, suggests self-determination which enables freedom to select and act according to one's will with independent thought and control over choices (Batey and Lewis, 1982; Rogers, 1983). Independence may be limited by circumstances and constraining factors (Jary and Jary, 1991; Wilkinson, 1997) but the belief in the concept of man as the author of his own destiny denies the limitations imposed by these circumstances (Kelly, 1981). Stevens (1984) has expressed the view that one is truly autonomous only when one is aware of the extent to which one is being determined by these external factors and there is evidence that this is acknowledged by nurses (Porter, 1992; Leddy and Pepper, 1993; Wilkinson, 1997). Hollis (1977), however, states the more extreme view that an assumption of complete freedom may actually indicate lack of autonomy.

There is ongoing debate about the interrelationship of the concepts of independence and autonomy. Wilkinson (1997) sees independence as the core theme of autonomy, which exists in varying degrees, whereas Mitchinson (1996) suggests that the two are entirely separate. Autonomous practice is synonymous with a degree of freedom to exercise professional judgement accorded to very few where, the practitioner defines, negotiates and develops professional practice. The key example quoted is the GP, whose role is seen to lack direct monitoring and supervision and who is accountable directly to the patient and the professional body for doctors, the General Medical Council (GMC), although this is likely to change with the new primary care trusts (PCTs), clinical governance and the National Institute of Clinical Excellence (NICE) (DOH, 1997c, 1998b, 1998d). In contrast, independent practice allows less freedom to define practice but practitioners are able to negotiate a degree of freedom within their prescribed role to practice independently of the direct supervision or monitoring of other practitioners or managers (Mitchinson 1996).

Mitchinson (1996) provides a concept analysis that identifies the critical defining attributes of the autonomous nurse as:

- Practises within a professional context which is self-regulating.
- Makes decisions based on professional judgement and has the ability to implement these within own sphere of practice.
- Cognisant with determining forces (bio-psycho-social) and has the knowledge to judge when these need to be accepted or challenged.

There is evidence to suggest that autonomous nurses experience greater satisfaction at work (McCloskey, 1990; Dwyer et al., 1992; Tingle, 1997). In further studies an association has been discovered between autonomy and the popularity of the workplace which has implications for nurse recruitment and retention (McCloskey, 1990; Dwyer et al., 1992; Hall, 1993; Tingle, 1997). There is also evidence to suggest that if colleagues in the workplace are perceived to be supportive of autonomy, higher competency results (Monninger, 1988; Dwyer et al., 1992).

Accountability and employment

The nurse, whether entrepreneur or employee, is accountable to the public and the professional body, the United Kingdom Central Council for nurses, midwives and health visitors (UKCC). The UKCC expects all registered nurses, midwives and health visitors to apply the principles inherent in the *Code of Professional Conduct* (UKCC, 1992a) and *The Scope of Professional Practice* (UKCC, 1992b), irrespective of where they are working and this clearly applies to those working in extended roles and within new initiatives such as nurse-led services. The Code (UKCC, 1992a) requires all registered practitioners to:

> Ensure that no action or omission on your part or within your sphere of responsibility is detrimental to the interests, condition or safety of patients and clients ... Acknowledge any limitations in your knowledge and competence and decline any duties or responsibilities unless able to perform them in a safe and skilled manner.
>
> (UKCC, 1992a:)

These principles are reinforced in *The Scope of Professional Practice* (UKCC, 1992b), which requires registered nurses to:

> Be satisfied that each aspect of practice is directed to meeting the needs and serving the interests of the patient or client ... Endeavour always to achieve, maintain and develop knowledge, skills and competence to respond to those needs and interests.
>
> (UKCC, 1992b:)

Knape (1999) also states that the need to maintain and develop professional knowledge and competence is addressed through clinical supervision and the UKCC's standards for continuing professional development (UKCC, 1994; UKCC 1999e; UKCC 2000b).

There appears to be much confusion, contradiction and a degree of difficulty in interpreting doctors' and nurses' accountability, particularly when *The Scope of Professional Practice* is compared with the statement of the GMC (1995) about the professional duties of doctors or the British Medical Association (BMA) (1996) document, *Protecting Patient Safety*, which gives guidelines on medical procedures performed by non-medically qualified health professionals (Dowling *et al.*, 1996; Tingle, 1997). For example, Clause 28 of the GMC (1995) statement views the doctor as maintaining overall responsibility for the care regime although aspects of that care may be delegated to a competent individual, whereas Clause 29 states that a doctor must not enable anyone who is not registered with the GMC to carry out tasks that require the knowledge and skills of a doctor. If Clause 29 were to be considered separately and literally, carrying out an extended nursing role would be impossible. The BMA guidelines (BMA, 1996) also strongly support the doctor as the manager and delegater of care. Early in 1999, the government announced radical plans to replace the UKCC and the national boards with a single UK-wide body (Clarke, 1999). It seems timely, perhaps, for a unified interprofessional body with the power to develop shared guidelines for medical, professions allied to medicine and nursing practice which would act as a single registration authority for health professionals. Failing this, it would be important for the three organizations to adopt a collaborative approach to develop a shared understanding of extended nursing roles and their interface with medical practice. There is resonance in the view that the duty of stakeholders, such as the UKCC, to collaborate should be reciprocal (While, 1999).

Nurses, like any health professionals, also owe their patients or clients an individual legal duty of care where a nurse is required to act in the best interests of the patient at all times. If employed, the nurse also owes this duty of care to fellow employees. Although claims for negligence against nurses are currently rare (Clarke, 1999), the claimant needs to prove the following in all cases of civil liability:

- That there was a *duty of care* between the parties.
- That there was a *breach of that duty.*
- That the breach *caused* the claimant harm (Clarke, 1999).

Breach of the duty of care is tested against the standard of care owed. For health professionals there is a specific test, the Bolam test, established in a civil trial in 1957 (2 All ER 118) (Clarke, 1999). Here, the court needs to prove that the standard of care is less than the standard of the ordinary skilled man exercising and professing to have that specialist skill (Clarke, 1999). It is not necessarily negligent if accepted practice is not followed as long as there is a body of competent professional opinion that supports the decision as reasonable in the circumstances (Clarke, 1999). However, it is certain that the more specialized the practitioner, the greater is the expected standard of care (Clarke, 1999). Another basic principle of the law of negligence is that the health professional can only take precautions against risks that were reasonably foreseeable (Clarke, 1999). The nurse, in the event of a claim, will therefore be judged against risks known at the time of the alleged incident (Clarke, 1999). This aspect also applies to omissions in communication with the patient or client. All personal injury claims are time-limited and must be instigated within three years of the date of the incident that caused harm except in the case of a child where the limitation period commences once the child reaches 18 (the Limitation Act 1980, Prescription and Limitation (Scotland) Act 1973, Limitation Order (NI) 1989). For those unaware that harm has occurred, the period commences from the date that they knew or should have known this and, for those with a disability, the period starts from the date of recovery if this occurs (Clarke, 1999). Some claims, however, may be extended at the discretion of the trial judge. In the case of a nurse working as an independent contractor in entrepreneurial situations, private indemnity insurance is therefore seen to be vitally important (RCN, 1997a).

Since the case of Cassidy versus the Ministry of Health in 1951 (2KB 293), the courts have also worked on the principle that, if the nurse is employed, the trust or health authority is also vicariously liable for any wrongful acts committed (Clarke, 1999). In this case, the claimant may choose to sue both the individual and the employer. It is more common for the employer to be sued as there are usually larger resources available to settle compensation claims (Clarke, 1999). The employer, however, retains the right to sue the employee as the contract of employment has an implied expectation that the employee will use reasonable skill and care in the performance of all duties, although this rarely happens (Dimond, 1994). In order to prove that the employer is vicariously liable, the claimant must prove:

- That the nurse was negligent.
- That the nurse was an employee.
- That the nurse was acting in the course of her employment. It is important to ascertain whether the act was authorized or prohibited by the employer. If the act is authorized then the employer is vicariously liable. However, if the employee is 'on a frolic of his own' and the act is completely unconnected with the job then the employer is not liable (Clarke, 1999).

Every trust also holds a non-delegable direct duty of care to its patients (primary liability) to employ competent staff with reasonable levels of supervision. This may mean that where a claimant cannot show negligence against an employee, it is still possible to take action against the employer (Clarke, 1999).

Three recent developments: clinical governance, the strategy designed to improve standards in the NHS; the formation of NICE, and the Commission for Health Improvement (CHI) will increase the accountability of nurses to patients, professional colleagues and each other (DOH, 1997c, 1998d). The main components of clinical governance are:

- Clear lines of responsibility and accountability for the overall quality of clinical care.
- A comprehensive programme of quality improvement systems.
- Clear policies aimed at managing risk and procedures for all professional groups to identify and address poor performance. The White Paper (DOH, 1997c) acknowledges that these arrangements will build on and strengthen the existing systems of professional self-regulation (Clarke, 1999).

A new framework for risk management in organizations, corporate governance, which includes professional liability, was introduced in 2000 as part of controls assurance within the NHS (DOH, 1999h).

Community changes

A range of changes in the organization of primary care has contributed to innovations in care delivery and new nursing roles. The most significant of these was the White Paper, *The New NHS – Modern and Dependable* (DOH, 1997c), which has led to the formation of PCGs to replace the old commissioning and fundholding groups (DOH, 1998b). These PCGs may elect to become primary care trusts (PCTs) following a public consultation process and, at Level 3, would be accountable to the health authority for commissioning care and, at Level 4, hold additional responsibility for the provision of community services for their population (DOH, 1999a). Trust status enables these organizations to flex people and resources to develop new services and new ways of working which may well lead to a proliferation of nurse-led services (DOH, 1999j, 1999k). First-wave PCTs became operational in April 2000 (DOH, 1999a). This White Paper also led to the establishment of NHS Direct, a new 24-hour telephone advice line for the public staffed by nurses. Three pilot helplines began in March 1998 with a view to having national coverage by the end of 2000 (DOH, 1999f, 1999g). Opportunities within NHS Direct and out-of-hours services or within general practice have enabled nurses to develop skills in telephone and face-to-face triage, with or without computer-assisted assessment, which have been well evaluated (Healy, 1997; Myers, 1997; Woodman, 1997; Jones et al., 1998; Lattimer, 2000). The current difficulties in recruiting and retaining GPs, particularly in inner city areas, have offered nurses the opportunity to develop innovative nurse-led community services through Primary Care Act (1997) pilot sites offering personal medical services (Gardner, 1998a; Chapple et al., 1999). One of these pilots uses a nurse to triage all consultations except where the patient expressly asks to see a doctor (Baraniak, 1999). A number of legislative problems have emerged within the first ten nurse-led personal medical services pilots (Gardner, 1998a):

- Nurses cannot sign sickness and death certificates.
- Nurses cannot section patients under the Mental Health Act 1984.
- Nurses cannot prescribe – except district nurses and health visitors (or practice nurses with one of these qualifications) and, for those who can, the formulary is very limited (mainly wound care products, urinary catheters and stoma appliances, elastic hosiery, simple analgesics, laxatives, some skin creams, head lice preparations).
- Health authorities and PCGs/PCTs are unable to allocate premises improvement grants to nurses.

These pilots have, in general, developed alternative services for vulnerable and socially excluded groups who often have difficulty accessing traditional services (Cantrill, 1997; McKeon, 1997; Gardner, 1998b; Chapple and Sergison, 1999). This fits with the government's plans to tackle health inequalities and social exclusion (DOH, 1998c, 1998f, 1998g, 1999d) formulated after publication of the Acheson Report (1997). A second wave of Primary Care Act pilot sites started in October 1999 and the NHS Executive was keen to encourage community nurses to bid, particularly if they could offer services which included evening and weekend surgeries (NHS Executive, 1998; Chapple and Sergison, 1999). On 13 April 1999, the Prime Minister announced the launch of primary care walk-in centres, and proposals for first-wave pilot sites had to be endorsed by PCGs before submission to the NHS Executive by the end of June 1999 (DOH, 1999e). Proposals were expected to fit a number of criteria and be co-located with other NHS services, such as accident and emergency (A&E) departments, minor injuries units, optical, pharmacy, dental or GP out-of-hours services, to test a range of service delivery configurations at the pilot phase. In time, these pilots may also enable further diversity of extended nursing roles.

Health action zones are pilot initiatives set up by the government in areas of deprivation to tackle health inequalities and create more integrated local care services through partnership working and breaking down organizational boundaries (DOH, 1998c; Evans and Robinson, 1999). Health action zones are testing grounds for new ideas and innovations expected to run for up to seven years which receive additional funding to support this local action to improve health. Strong links are expected to develop between the health action zone and local three-year HImPs (DOH, 1998f, 1998g, 1999l). There are now 26 health action zones (11 first-wave in 1998 and 15 second-wave in 1999) in areas with significant health needs in England. Two of the core principles of the health action zone are involvement of local people in planning the services and involvement of all staff in strategy development. These areas will provide opportunities for new ways of working and extended nursing roles across boundaries and, for those areas not designated as health action zones, opportunities to learn from the pilot areas through information-sharing and the rigorous evaluation that is expected in each. Healthy living centres and networks are also being established to complement existing provision with £300 million of National Lottery funding through the New Opportunities Fund (DOH, 1999m). These initiatives are designed to improve health and reduce health inequalities through local community action and are seen to be complementary to *Our Healthier Nation* (DOH, 1998c) and local HImPs. Areas with health action zones in place and those with urban degeneration or rural deprivation are seen to be particularly rich testing beds for new ideas. It is expected that healthy living centres will demonstrate new ways of working across current boundaries (voluntary, private and public) and innovative approaches to providing opportunities for people to improve their health and well-being. Nurses, as well as other health professionals, may also have opportunities to develop different roles within these centres.

Professional changes with implications for autonomy

Apart from the guidance from the UKCC about the scope of professional practice and the *Code of Professional Conduct* (UKCC, 1992a, 1992b, 1996a) to which all nurses must adhere, there has been ongoing debate about the constituents of advanced nursing practice and the similarities and differences between clinical specialist and nurse practitioner roles and whether or not there is, in fact, any difference between the two (Castledine, 1995; McGee *et al.*, 1996; UKCC, 1996a; McGee and Castledine, 1999). In 1994, the UKCC stated its commitment to developing the concept of advanced practice and outlined the consultation process that would be involved (UKCC, 1996b, 1997a). This strategy consisted of three main stages: a listening exercise involving written submissions and telephone or face-to-face interviews; a seminar conducted with the four national Boards, and a consultative conference with 100 participants to test the views and opinions gained. The outcome was that the UKCC decided that explicit standards for advanced practice should not be set but there was a strong consensus for the need to retain the concept of advancing practice. However, in December 1997, the UKCC released a further paper with proposals to develop a framework for specialist practice, which embraced both nurse practitioners and clinical nurse specialists within it (UKCC, 1997b). In October 1998, the UKCC released a consultation document with seven questions on its proposals for regulation of advanced practice within the post-registration regulatory framework (UKCC, 1998). Analysis of the questionnaire responses resulted in the production of a draft standard and descriptor for a higher level of practice (UKCC, 1999a, 1999b). This development was reinforced by the view from the report (JM Consulting, 1999) on the Nurses, Midwives and Health Visitors Act (1997) that the new nursing and midwifery council proposed by the government could define standards in terms of outcomes for an entry on the register which would denote achievement of a higher level of practice. In order to be recognized as practising at a higher level, nurses would need to achieve all the criteria under each of the following practice areas of the generic draft standard developed:

- Providing effective healthcare.
- Improving quality and health outcomes.
- Evaluation and research.
- Leading and developing practice.
- Innovation and changing practice.
- Developing self and others.
- Working across professional and organizational boundaries.

Feedback about the standard has been very positive and the UKCC has now commissioned a series of pilot studies by the City and Guilds Affinity involving 300 nurses, midwives and health visitors to test the modified standard's robustness and applicability to all health care settings (UKCC, 1999c, 2000). These practitioners are required to develop a portfolio of evidence of their competence to practise which will be verified in the workplace before being assessed by a panel which comprises an individual from the same profession as the practitioner, a lay member representing the interests of patients and clients and two practitioners, one from a different and one from the same profession as the individual but both working in a similar area of practice (UKCC 1999d, 2000). Although it is to be applauded that these negotiations to identify advanced practice have involved in-depth consultation with practitioners, health professionals, a range of organizations and the public, it is regrettable that it has taken almost 16 years since the first introduction of nurse practitioners to the UK and six years since the statement regarding specialist practice was published by the UKCC (1994) for this point in the process to be reached. This has resulted in much confusion for professionals and the public and has delayed protection of the public.

The UKCC's higher level of practice framework fits coherently with the government's proposals to develop nurse consultant posts to provide a clinical career structure for nurses and retain experienced and senior practitioners within practice (DOH, 1999c, 1999i). These posts have also been designed to strengthen nursing leadership and provide better outcomes for patients by improving the quality of services (DOH, 1999h) and are structured around four core functions which are closely interrelated:

- An expert function.
- A professional leadership and consultancy function.
- An education, training and development function.
- A practice and service development, research and evaluation function.

It has been recognized that the amount of time spent on each core function will differ from post to post and with time as needs change but nurse consultants must spend at least 50% of their time working directly with patients, clients or communities (DOH, 1999i). The Department of Health (DOH, 1999i) has stated that although the UKCC's higher level of practice standard will provide a very helpful eligibility criterion, not all those who are accredited as working at this advanced level will become consultant practitioners, although it will be adopted by the NHS as a necessary condition of employment. However, it is anticipated that proposals to establish such posts will include an indication of willingness to participate in the further development and piloting of the UKCC standard (DOH, 1999i). The term 'nurse [or midwife or health visitor] consultant' therefore denotes an NHS employment category. There were to be 141 new posts in the first wave of nurse consultants in April 2000 and, of these, it was anticipated that seven would be directly employed in primary care (*Practice Nurse*, 2000). These include three posts in walk-in centres, one in a PCT in Essex to develop the public health agenda and needs assessment, and one attached to Hillingdon Health Authority to provide clinical leadership for nurses working in GP practices and to undertake a clinical caseload within a personal medical services pilot. There are plans to more than double the number of nurse consultants within a year (DOH, 2000c). Although most practitioners appear to have welcomed this innovation, there has been a suggestion that it is a cheap political stunt to boost poll ratings (Duffin, 2000).

Nurse prescribing will assist in the development of extended nursing roles once the limited drug formulary is extended and the professional groups widened to include other nurses apart from those eligible to prescribe at present, namely district nurses, health visitors and practice nurses with either of these qualifications (DOH, 1989, 1999b). In March 2000, Health Ministers confirmed in a press release (2000/0146) that the Crown Report to extend prescribing to other groups had been accepted (DOH, 1999b, 2000a). Two groups of prescribers have been identified, *supplementary* (dependent, including district nurses and health visitors) and *independent* (responsible for assessment and clinical management of patients with undiagnosed conditions, including prescribing). Until the Medicines Act 1968 and other relevant legislation is changed, nurse practitioners who are not currently legal prescribers may administer medicines under patient group directions (group protocols) designed for specific groups of patients with specified problems or clinical conditions and ratified by a doctor (or dentist), the health authority (or PCG as a subcommittee of the health authority), NHS Trust or PCT and local prescribing committees (DOH, 1998e, 2000b; MCA, 2000). It is expected that the clinical governance lead for the organization concerned will also be involved in this process. The guidance states that most prescribing should be undertaken on a named-patient basis and patient group directions are seen to be most useful for a limited range of situations, including minor injury units, A&E departments, walk-in centres, family planning clinics and for immunization programmes (DOH, 2000a). However, for nurses working in extended roles, Cullen (2000) cautions that such protocols may actually inhibit rather than enhance prescribing ability and associated skills.

In 1999, the Audit Commission published a report (Audit Commission, 1999) which highlighted deficiencies in current district nurse provision as services endeavour to cope with increasing demand due in part to the shifting of care from secondary to primary providers and earlier discharge of patients from hospital. The strategy for nursing, *Making a Difference* (DOH, 1999c), also identifies the potential for closer integration between district nurses and practice nurses to increase flexibility, efficiency and responsiveness of services. It will require the support of the different community nurse employers, some of whom may be resistant to these changes. It is possible that when PCTs employ all community nurses, including practice nurses, closer integration will result. This integration may give scope for self-managed nursing teams as well as innovative models of care delivery utilizing the key skills of all members of the team and the advanced skills of those working in an extended role, which are not necessarily maximized within conventional services. One personal medical services pilot in the Black Country, the Aladin Project, has demonstrated the positive benefits to practitioners and patients of this method of skill-mixing and integration (Bradbury *et al.*, 1998). Other studies reinforce these benefits (Black and Hagel, 1997; Godfrey *et al.*, 1997; Jenkins-Clarke *et al.*, 1997).

Making a Difference (DOH, 1999c) also suggests that every NHS organization should use clinical supervision and statutory midwifery supervision to help identify, support and develop nurse, midwife and health visitor leaders and potential leaders. There is also a wealth of evidence to show the positive benefits of clinical supervision in relation to professional development and quality of care through reflection on practice (Damant *et al.*, 1994; Kohner, 1994; Palmer *et al.*, 1994; Sams, 1996; Twinn *et al.*, 1996; Gastrell and Edwards, 1998; Cheater, 1999; Dunn *et al.*, 1999; Proctor *et al.*, 1999). It has also been suggested that clinical supervision should be an essential component for clinical governance frameworks in primary care, particularly where practitioners work in isolation (Aitkin *et al.*, 1993; Cook, 1996; Cheater, 1999; Dunn *et al.*, 1999; Hale 1999; Styles *et al.*, 1999). It appears from the evidence that many nurses using extended skills in primary care work within general practices as nurse practitioners and it seems important to support development of their skills and roles through clinical supervision.

One of the difficulties for nurses employed in general practices may be persuading GPs of the merits of such a system, particularly if it removes them from patient contact during working hours. It is regrettable that clinical supervision, at the present time, is voluntary and not mandatory when such overwhelming evidence confirms its benefits for professional practice. A mandatory requirement would also enable these nurses employed by practices to participate in supervision activity while employed rather than in their own time and ensure its uptake so that it becomes an integral part of clinical governance. As interdisciplinary education becomes more widespread and role boundaries more blurred, it would be helpful for nurses working in advanced roles to participate in group supervision activities with medical practitioners. It is to be expected that some time would be needed during the initial forming process of such a group for trust to develop between the different professions. However, this model of supervision may maximize collaboration, promote shared understanding and mutual respect and disseminate good practice, as well as enhancing professional development.

Educational developments

The English National Board (ENB) for nursing, midwifery and health visiting launched a framework for continuing professional education and the higher award in 1992 which aimed to support excellence in practice by offering a flexible and coherent system for continuing education, thus enabling practitioners to access relevant learning opportunities and so demonstrate expert practice supported by relevant professional knowledge (ENB, 1991). The framework and higher award are available at Board-approved educational institutes throughout England and 80 outline curricula are now available covering the range of specialities and more designed by local institutes to meet specific local needs (ENB, 1997, 2000a). The framework appears to be based on an effective partnership between practitioners, education and managers to ensure that education is service-led, meets the need for quality of care and promotes the philosophy of lifelong learning (ENB, 1995). Similar processes exist within the areas covered by the Boards for Northern Ireland, Scotland and Wales.

A research team from the University of Sheffield has recently completed an evaluation of the implementation of this framework and higher award highlighting detailed concerns and recommended changes, which will be taken into account in the ENB review of post-registration programmes (ENB, 2000b). However, some of the recommendations are dependent on the final decision about the UKCC's higher level of practice and the implementation of changes arising from the review of the Nurses, Midwives and Health Visitors Act 1997. There is an anomaly in this situation in that some of the courses offered to nurses developing extended practice, although approved by a higher education institute, are not necessarily approved by the ENB and therefore do not attract the ENB Higher Award. One such course, the first nationally, is that organized by the Institute of Advanced Education at the Royal College of Nursing, which is now franchised to other universities, where successful candidates are awarded solely the RCN Nurse Practitioner

Professional Award. Conversely, the RCN Diploma, considered to be a quality marker for nurse practitioner preparation, is also only available at a small number of higher education institutes. It is important, for the future, to rationalize this system so that it becomes universal and accessible in a similar way to advanced practice, thus ensuring clarity, equality of opportunity and preventing confusion among practitioners. It is also important that nurses undertaking extended roles are able to access courses at Masters level and above (Feeney, 1999).

Little research has so far been undertaken about the courses offered in preparation for nurse practitioner practice in the UK. However, Andrewes *et al.* (1999) undertook a qualitative research study through individual and focus group interviews, with students who had completed the diploma-level nurse practitioner foundation course at Bournemouth University. This was to ascertain the impact of this course, identify the nursing components of the role and the elements that constitute the expanded responsibility of the qualified nurse in order to inform the degree-level course components. The outcomes identified a number of changes necessary to prepare the nurse practitioner for the future, including an applied pharmacology and pathophysiology module to enable administration of drugs under protocol, a clinical intervention unit, an enhanced unit to enable students to understand the skills and knowledge required to undertake health assessment and a mandatory open day for students and those supporting them to discuss support in practice and clarification of the future role students will be expected to undertake: a pre-course learning contract is now agreed by the nurse, the manager and mentor.

Nurse practitioner roles

HISTORICAL PERSPECTIVES IN THE USA AND THE UK

In America, where nurse practitioners have been practising since the mid-1960s, most of the evidence in the literature focuses on the role of the family nurse practitioner within primary care in relation to urban populations. It is estimated that there are now more than 50 000 nurse practitioners (Ashburner *et al.*, 1997) and their development has flourished due to a shortage of physicians in general medical practice (Rogers, 1977; Sultz, 1983). A meta-analysis by Brown and Grimes (1995) revealed that 12 randomized, controlled trials on the effectiveness of nurse practitioners in primary care in North America have occurred. The results show some evidence of the positive effects of nurse practitioners in relation to patient compliance with treatment. However, as the literature reviewed relates to studies undertaken in 1992, the results are somewhat outdated and no further systematic review appears to have been undertaken since that time.

The rural role appears to have developed in America in the last ten years in response to a care gap within the provision of health services, and a wealth of anecdotal evidence for the role exists in professional journals (Schmidt *et al.*, 1995; Vrabec, 1995; Pierce and Luikart, 1996; Alexy and Elnitsky, 1996). Rural areas, like inner city areas, were unpopular sites for medical practices within the private system of health care provision because of their professional and personal remoteness and the sparse population (Ashburner *et al.*, 1997). The rural family nurse practitioner appears to work in isolation as the rural health care system is often limited or absent. The models that have developed include mobile clinics to meet the needs of farm workers (Stein, 1993), the rural elderly (Garrett, 1995) and community-based health care units (Hopkins, 1993).

In contrast, the nurse practitioner role in the UK appears to have evolved from the practice nurse role (Greenfield, 1992; Rowley, 1994; Atkin and Lunt, 1995; Hunter and MacAuley, 1996). Barbara Stilwell is the name synonymous with the role in primary care in the UK (Bryer, 1994). She worked alongside two GPs in Birmingham offering an alternative service focusing on prevention of disease and social problems rather than a medical curative model (Stilwell *et al.*, 1987; Salisbury and Tettersall, 1988). The other pioneer, also working in inner city areas, was Burke-Masters who studied the role in relation to the homeless (Burke-Masters, 1986). Salisbury and Tettersall (1988) also looked at the nurse practitioner role as an alternative to the doctor in the practice but, although it was intended that the workload was shared equally, this did not happen and the GP workload remained the same.

Fawcett-Hennessey (1991) described the characteristics of the nurse practitioner as:

- Providing choice for patients.
- Having diagnostic and prescribing power.
- Having authority for referral.
- Offering more personal attention and time during consultation.
- Having a particular interest in counselling and health education.

The RCN has a more extensive definition of a nurse practitioner, agreed by Council in 1997, and widely accepted by nurse practitioners as the constituents of their role:

- Makes professionally autonomous decisions for which s/he has sole responsibility.
- Receives patients and clients with undifferentiated and undiagnosed problems. Assessment of their health care needs is made based on highly developed nursing knowledge and skills. This includes special skills, such as physical examination, not usually undertaken by nurses.
- Screens patients and clients for disease risk factors and early signs of illness.
- Develops with the patient or client a nursing care plan with an emphasis on preventive measures.
- Provides counselling and health education.
- Has the authority to admit or discharge patients and clients from own caseload and refer them to other health care providers as appropriate.

The shift of workload from secondary to primary care has focused attention on the potential of nurse practitioners as promoters of health and as the providers of services to people who are not receiving health care at the social frontiers (Jordan, 1992; Jackson, 1995; Chambers, 1998). The UKCC (1996b) has stated that nurse practitioners in primary care, where the nurse substitutes for the doctor, are not felt to meet the criteria of advanced practice but would meet the criteria of specialist practice. Advanced practice is seen to be innovative and developed at the cutting edge and would therefore apply to a new service or method of working.

Evaluation of the role of nurse practitioners in terms of clinical and cost effectiveness has been seen to be critical to their development in primary care (Ashburner et al., 1997). One of the first rigorous research studies producing evidence that suggested that nurse practitioners could be as effective as medical colleagues was the Burlington Randomized Trial which involved 1500 families in Ontario, Canada (Sackett et al., 1974). Patients were followed up for one year and the researchers could find no difference in outcome measures of physical, emotional and social function between those receiving nurse and those receiving physician care. Patient satisfaction was also equally high within the two groups. In this country, the first research commissioned by the NHS Executive in 1995, evaluated nurse practitioner projects at ten different sites, six of which were in primary care and found that the outcomes were very positive for nurse practitioner services (Coopers and Lybrand, 1995).

The outcomes were defined in terms of access to services, costs of services and impact on waiting times. Results showed reduced waiting times and similar or reduced costs for comparable services; however, comparison between these services and conventional ones is difficult.

A two-year review by Touche Ross (1994) of nurse practitioner projects in south London was also very positive of the role but the review is seen to be somewhat descriptive. Fall et al. (1997), through the use of a questionnaire, also conducted an evaluation of a nurse-led ear care service in Rotherham and Barnsley using a control group of similar patients treated by standard practice. Results showed that the nurses trained in ear care reduced costs, GP workload and the use of systemic antibiotics.

The evaluation, using a qualitative case study approach, of a nurse-led personal medical services pilot scheme set up following the 1997 NHS (Primary Care) Act, which was undertaken by the National Primary Care Research and Development Centre at the University of Manchester, found that:

- The service provides a point of access, continuity and stability in a deprived area.
- The service takes an holistic approach to health taking account of emotional, social and health needs.
- Patient satisfaction with the nurse-led service is high. This was found to be the most significant and consistent finding and relied in part on the opportunity to form relationships with health professionals who provided continuity of care.
- Patients value the excellent communication they have with the professionals.
- Nurse-led schemes provide a viable option for areas where GPs are hard to recruit (Chapple et al., 1999).

A recent multicentred, randomized, controlled trial of nurse practitioner versus GP care for 1368 patients requesting same-day consultations in primary care also supports the wider acceptance of the nurse practitioner role, in that patients, particularly children, were more satisfied with the care, resolution of symptoms and concerns did not differ and the number of prescriptions issued, investigations ordered, referrals to secondary care and re-attendances were similar between the two groups (Kinnersley et al., 2000).

However, patients managed by the NPs reported receiving significantly more information about their illnesses and, in all but one practice, their consultations were longer (ten minutes instead of eight minutes).

A further randomized controlled trial comparing cost-effectiveness of GPs and nurse practitioners in primary care undertaken with 1292 patients in 20 practices has also demonstrated that the clinical care and health service costs of the two types of practitioner is similar but that if the nurse practitioners were able to maintain the benefits to patients while reducing their return consultation rate (37.2% versus 24.8%) or shortening the consultation time (11 minutes plus 1.33 minutes per patient waiting for prescriptions to be signed versus seven minutes) then they could be more cost-effective than GPs (Venning et al., 2000). There is a view that nurse practitioners may not really be needed in primary care as 17% of consultations can be completely delegated and effectively managed by practice and other community nurses and 39% have delegatable elements (Jenkins-Clarke et al., 1997). However, one-third of this delegation needed to be to an enhanced team. A further rigorous multicentre study with 1815 patients in five south London practices where patients with minor illnesses were randomly assigned to either GPs or specially trained (three-month part-time degree-level course) practice nurses appears to support this view in that patients were significantly more satisfied with their consultations with practice nurses, the patients seen were also managed without input from the GP and a similar number of prescriptions were issued by the two groups (Shum et al., 2000). Consultations with the practice nurse were marginally longer (approximately ten minutes) than with the GP (eight minutes).

A scoping exercise by the Centre for Health Planning and Management at Keele University has discovered difficulties in assessing just how widespread nurse practitioners are in primary care in the UK given the issues surrounding definition – clinical specialist / nurse practitioner / advanced nurse practitioner (Healy, 1996; Castledine, 1997) and the methodological means of collecting the data, which in this case was questionnaires sent to individual health authorities (Ashburner et al., 1997). It also appears that many nurse practitioners have developed roles which liaise or work across existing boundaries, such as primary and secondary care and this makes classification difficult (Read, 1995; Ashburner et al., 1997). McGee et al. (1996) surveyed 230 trusts but were unable to identify any advanced nurse practitioners in primary care. It is possible that some innovations were missed, for example, in fund holding practices as this survey was completed by the chair and chief nurse in each Trust.

DIVERSITY OF EXTENDED ROLES

Since the early 1990s, there is evidence to show a diverse proliferation of nurse-led acute services where the nurse works autonomously to provide an alternative service for patients. These services relate to areas such as accident and emergency (A&E) (Freeman *et al.*, 1999), minor injuries (Baker, 1993; Dolan *et al.*, 1997), chronic diseases such as rheumatology (Hill, 1997), out-patient clinics (Phillips, 1995; Mackie, 1996) and nurse-led beds (Griffiths, 1995). Ryan (1997) describes a nurse-led drug monitoring service for rheumatology patients. Only two of these roles in the UK appear to have been rigorously evaluated: Hill's (1994) study of the nurse-led rheumatology service and a study by Whitehouse (1994) relating to the nurse practitioner role with patients with Parkinson's disease.

In Hill's (1994) study, 70 patients were randomized to receive care either from the nurse practitioner or the consultant rheumatologist. Patients were followed up for one year, receiving six sessions from the same professional. The satisfaction scores increased for the nurse practitioner at the end of the study period but remained the same for the consultant. The nurse practitioner saw only eight patients in a four-hour period, whereas the consultant saw 17. The length of the consultation would have undoubtedly affected patient satisfaction.

Community nurse-led services have been slower to develop, although the first appears to have been the service for the homeless developed by Burke-Masters (1986). The nurse practitioner role in GP practices now seems to be well-established, although the majority of the published evidence appears to be anecdotal. Expansion of the nurse practitioner role in the community also appears to be emerging in health visiting and mental health (Torn and McNichol, 1996; Obeid, 1998).

The future

Although there are a number of potential pitfalls that have already been described in some detail in this chapter, overall, the next decade heralds a wonderful time of opportunity for nursing and primary care. The formation of PCTs with enhanced ability to flex people and resources will ensure that the NHS is more responsive and that there is the will to develop new ways of working. There also appears to be political will to liberate nurses' talents and the Health Secretary, Alan Milburn, has just unveiled a ten-point challenge on nursing skills to be implemented in every part of the NHS (DOH, 2000c):

1. To order diagnostic investigations such as pathology tests and X-rays.
2. To make and receive referrals – direct to, for example, therapists or pain consultants.
3. To admit and discharge patients for specified conditions and with agreed protocols.
4. To manage their own patient caseloads, for example, for diabetes and rheumatology.
5. To run their own clinics, for example, for ophthalmology or dermatology.

6. To prescribe medicines and treatment.
7. To carry out a wide range of resuscitation procedures such as defibrillation and intubation.
8. To perform minor surgery and outpatient procedures.
9. To use computerized decision support to triage patients to the most appropriate health professional.
10. To take a lead in the way local services are organized and run.

Nurses working in extended roles have already shown that they can manage effectively, without need for referral, 70–88% of patient consultations currently undertaken by GPs (Richardson and Maynard, 1995; Marsh and Dawes, 1995; Reveley, 1998). Medical colleagues are divided about the advantages and disadvantages of a salaried GP service and it will be interesting to see the outcomes in terms of clinical and cost-effectiveness and quality of care if the UK moves to a similar model to the USA where the majority of primary care is undertaken by advanced nurse practitioners and the GP is locality-based as a specialist resource for referral of patients with complex or uncertain diagnoses. This would mirror secondary care where the consultant is available for specialist advice. This view is not about interprofessional power struggles, although individuals may feel threatened (Kernick, 1998); it is about collaboration and partnership, maximizing the skills and abilities of each member of the primary health care team through skill-mix in order to utilize precious resources effectively for the highest possible quality of care. If primary care becomes nurse-led, the nurse practitioner role would not be seen to be a doctor-substitute or doctor's assistant and would therefore fit with the UKCC definition of advanced practice (UKCC, 1996a). The other area where development possibilities exist is with the socially excluded and it would be important to build on the vanguard services that already exist in some areas and address the issues associated with unmet health needs while providing services for these groups that they will wish to access. These suggestions would need changes in the law to enable, for example, nurses leading services to prescribe a broad range of medicines, to be able to certify sickness and death and for patients to be able register with nurses (or with localities which may enhance flexibility and patient choice of where they access services) (RCN, 1997b). Williams and Sibbald (1999), however, caution that any shift of health care work from one professional group to another with consequent change of roles and identities creates a culture of uncertainty which has implications for the future of primary health care nursing. It is to be hoped that any such developments in primary care will ensure that people receive the highest quality health care when and where they need it.

References

Acheson Report. (1997) *Independent inquiry into inequalities in health*. London: The Stationery Office.
Aitkin, K., Lunt, N., Parker, G. *et al*. (1993) *Nurses count: a national census of practice nurses*. York: Social Policy Research Unit.

Alexy, B. and Elnitsky, C. (1996) Community outreach: rural mobile clinic. *Journal of Nursing Administration*, 26: 38–42.

Andrewes, C., Potter, P., Galvin, K., *et al.* (1999) *The changing nurse: NPs' perspectives on their role and education*. Bournemouth: Institute of Health and Community Studies, Bournemouth University.

Ashburner, L. Birch, K. Latimer, J. and Scrivens, E. (1997) *Nurse practitioners in primary care: the extent of practice and research*. Keele: Centre for Health Planning and Management, Keele University.

Atkin, K and Lunt, N. (1995) *Nurse in practice York*: Social Policy Research Unit, University of York.

Audit Commission. (1999) *First assessment: a review of district nursing services in England and Wales*. London: Audit Commission.

Baker, B. (1993) Model methods. *Nursing Times*, 89: 33–5.

Baraniak, C. (1999) Nurse in the pilot seat. *Primary Health Care*, 9: 6–8.

Batey, M.V. and Lewis F.M. (1982) Clarifying autonomy and accountability in nursing service: part 1. *Journal of Nursing Administration*, 12: 13–18.

Black, S. and Hagel, D. (1997) Developing an integrated nursing team approach. *Health Visitor*, 69: 280–3.

British Medical Association (BMA) (1996) *Protecting patient safety: medical procedures performed by non-medically qualified health professionals*. London: BMA.

Bradbury, P., Davidson, J., Macfarlane, L. and Werhun, P. (1998) Revolution in the black country. *Primary Health Care*, 8: 14–16.

Brown, A. and Grimes, D. (1995) A meta-analysis of nurse practitioners and nurse midwives in primary care. *Nursing Research*, 44: 332–9.

Bryar, R. (1994) An examination for new roles in the primary health care team. *Journal of Interprofessional Care*, 8: 73–5.

Burke-Masters, B. (1986) The autonomous nurse practitioner – an answer to the chronic problem of primary care. *Lancet*, 1: 1266.

Cantrill, P. (1997) Primary care scheme aims for partnership in practice. *Nursing Times*, 93: 56–7.

Castledine, G. (1995) Defining specialist nursing. *British Journal of Nursing*, 4: 264–5.

Castledine, G. (1997) The abuse of specialist titles must stop. *British Journal of Nursing*, 6: 1137.

Chambers, N. (1998) *Nurse practitioners in primary care*. Abingdon: Radcliffe Medical Press.

Chapple, A., Macdonald, W., Rogers, A. and Sergison, M. (1999) *Can nurses replace GPs? An evaluation of a nurse-led personal medical services pilot scheme*. Executive Summary 12. Manchester: National Primary Care Research and Development Centre, University of Manchester.

Chapple, A. and Sergison, M. (1999) Challenging tradition. *Nursing Times*, 95: 32–3.

Cheater, F.M. (1999) *An evaluation of the clinical supervision scheme for Leicestershire practice nurses*. Leicester: Department of General Practice and Primary Health Care, University of Leicester.

Clarke, A. (1999) *Community nurses and the law*. London: Community Practitioners and Health Visitors Association.

Cook, R. (1996) Clinical supervision: a talking shop? *Practice Nursing*, 7: 12–13.

Coopers and Lybrand. (1995) *Nurse practitioner evaluation project. Final report: executive summary*. Uxbridge: Coopers and Lybrand.

Cullen, C. (2000) Autonomy and the nurse practitioner. *Journal of the RCN Nurse Practitioner Association*, 54–6.

Damant, M., Martin, C., Openshaw, S. (1994) *Practice nursing stability and change.* London: Mosby.

Department of Health (DOH). (1989) *Report of the advisory group on nurse prescribing (Crown Report).* London: DOH.

Department of Health (DOH). (1995) *GP's out of hours services.* FHSL (95)68. London: DOH.

Department of Health (DOH). (1997a) *National Health Service (Primary Care) Act 1997.* London: The Stationery Office.

Department of Health (DOH). (1997b) *Implementing the Primary Care Act personal medical services pilots.* MISC (97) 86. London: DOH.

Department of Health (DOH). (1997c) *The new NHS – modern and dependable.* London: The Stationery Office.

Department of Health (DOH). (1998a) *Personal medical services pilots second wave.* HSC 1998/176. London: DOH.

Department of Health (DOH). (1998b) *The new NHS – modern and dependable establishing primary care groups.* HSC 1998/065. London: DOH.

Department of Health (DOH). (1998c) *Our healthier nation: a contract for health.* London: The Stationery Office.

Department of Health (DOH). (1998d) *A first class service – quality in the new NHS.* London: The Stationery Office.

Department of Health (DOH). (1998e) *Review of prescribing, supply and administration of medicines: a report on the supply and administration of medicines under group protocol.* London: DOH.

Department of Health (DOH). (1998f) *Health improvement programmes planning for better health and better health care.* HSC 1998/167. London: DOH.

Department of Health (DOH). (1998g) *Better health and better health care implementing 'The new NHS' and 'Our healthier nation'.* HSC 1998/021. London: DOH.

Department of Health (DOH). (1999a) *Primary care trusts: consultation on proposals to establish a primary care trust.* HSC 1999/207. London: DOH.

Department of Health (DOH). (1999b) *Review of prescribing, supply and administration of medicines.* Led by Dr June Crown. London: DOH.

Department of Health (DOH). (1999c) *Making a difference: strengthening the nursing, midwifery and health visiting contribution to health and healthcare.* London: The Stationery Office.

Department of Health (DOH). (1999d) *Saving lives: our healthier nation.* London: The Stationery Office.

Department of Health (DOH). (1999e) *NHS primary care walk-in centres selection of pilot sites for 1999/2000.* HSC 1999/116. London: DOH.

Department of Health (DOH). (1999f) *NHS Direct final stage of the roll-out.* HSC 1999/028. London: DOH.

Department of Health (DOH). (1999g) *NHS Direct and primary care – liability issues.* HSC 1999/235. London: DOH.

Department of Health (DOH). (1999h) *Governance in the new NHS controls assurance statements 1999/2000 risk management and organisational controls.* HSC 1999/123. London: DOH.

Department of Health (DOH). (1999i) *Nurse, midwife and health visitor consultants: establishing posts and making appointments.* HSC 1999/217. London: DOH.

Department of Health (DOH). (1999j) *Development of human resource management practices for primary care trusts.* Misc (99)30 London: DOH.

Department of Health (DOH). (1999k) *Minimum requirements to address human resource issues in primary care trusts.* HSC 1999/207. London: DOH.

Department of Health (DOH). (1999l) *Saving lives: our healthier nation White Paper and reducing health inequalities: a action report.* HSC 1999/152. London: DOH.

Department of Health (DOH). (1999m) *Healthy living centres.* HSC 1999/008. London: DOH.

Department of Health. (DOH). (2000a) *Go-ahead for plans to allow nurses to prescribe more medicines (changes to expand nurses jobs in A&E and NHS walk-in centres).* Final Press Release 2000/0146. London: DOH.

Department of Health (DOH). (2000b) *Patient group directions.* Draft HSC. London: DOH.

Department of Health (DOH). (2000c) Health Secretary lays out plans to liberate nurses talents: new vision to transform the NHS for nurses. Press Release 2000/0209. London: DOH.

Dimond, B. (1994) Legal aspects of role expansion. In: Hunt, G. and Wainwright, P. (eds) *Expanding the role of the nurse: the scope of professional practice.* Oxford: Blackwell.

Dolan, B., Dale, J. and Morley, V. (1997) Nurse practitioners: the role in A&E and primary care. *Nursing Standard,* 11: 33–8.

Dowling, S., Martin, R., Skidmore, P. *et al.* (1996) Nurses taking on junior doctors work: a confusion of accountability. *British Medical Journal,* 312: 1211–14.

Dwyer, D. J., Schwartz, R. J., Skidmore, P. *et al.* (1992) Decision making, autonomy in nursing. Journal of Nursing Administration, 22: 17–23.

Duffin, C. (2000) Will our paths cross? *Nursing Standard,* 14: 12–13.

Dunn, L., Banga, S., Downing, K. et al. (1999) Reap the benefits of clinical supervision. *Practice Nurse,* 18: 19–22.

English National Board (ENB). (1991) *Framework for continuing professional education for nurses, midwives and health visitors.* London: ENB.

English National Board (ENB). (1995) *Creating lifelong learners: partnerships for care, guidelines for the implementation of the UKCC's standards for education and practice following registration.* London: ENB.

English National Board (ENB). (1997) *Standards for approval of higher education institutions and programmes.* London: ENB.

English National Board (ENB). (2000a) *Continuing professional education.* London: ENB (see website at http://193.63.22.46/partners/enb/continue.html).

English National Board (ENB). (2000b) *ENB news: working together.* 35 London: ENB.

Evans, S. and Robinson, M. (1999) Take action to tackle health inequalities. *Practice Nurse,* 17: 218–22.

Fall, M., Walters, S., Read, S. *et al.* (1997) An evaluation of a nurse-led ear care service in primary care: benefits and costs. *British Journal of General Practice,* 47: 699–703.

Fawcett-Hennessey, A. (1991) The British scene. In: Salvage, J. (ed.) *Nurse practitioners: working for change in primary care.* London: King's Fund.

Feeney, J. (1999) Nurse practitioners in general practice. *Practice Nursing,* 10: 16–18.

Freeman, G.K., Meakin, R.P., Lawrenson, R.A. *et al.* (1999) Primary care units in A&E departments in North Thames in the 1990s: initial experience and future implications. *British Journal of General Practice,* 49: 107–10.

Gardner, L. (1998a) Nurse-led primary care act pilot schemes: threat or opportunity? *Nursing Times*, 94: 52–3.

Gardner, L. (1998b) Does nurse-led care mean second-class care? *Nursing Times*, 94: 50-1.

Garrett, D.K. (1995) Mobile access: opening health care doors. *Nurse Management*, 26: 29, 31–3.

Gastrell, P. and Edwards, J. (ed.) (1998) *Community health nursing frameworks for practice*. London: Bailliere Tindall.

General Medical Council (GMC) (1995) *Duties of a doctor, good medical practice*. London, GMC.

Godfrey, E., Rink, P. and Ross, F. (1997) Measuring the workload of an integrated nursing team in general practice. *British Journal of Community Health Nursing*, 2: 350–5.

Greenfield, S. (1992) Nurse practitioners and the changing face of general practice. In: Loveridge, R. and Starkey, K. (eds) *Continuity and crisis in the NHS*. Milton Keynes: Open University Press.

Griffiths, P. (1995) Evaluation of nurse-led in-patient care. *Nursing Times*, 25: 34–7.

Hale, C. (1999) Providing support for nurses in general practice through clinical supervision. A key element of the clinical governance framework. *Journal of Clinical Governance*, 7: 162–5.

Hall, S. (1993) The shock of the new. *Nursing Times*, 89: 63.

Healy, P. (1996) Confusion reigns over nurse practitioners. *Nursing Standard*, 11: 13.

Healy, P. (1997) Ringing the changes. *Nursing Standard*, 11: 14.

Hill, J. (1994) An evaluation of the effectiveness, safety and acceptability of a nurse practitioner in a rheumatology outpatient clinic. *British Journal of Rheumatology*, 33: 283–8.

Hill, J. (1997) Patient satisfaction in a nurse-led rheumatology clinic. *Journal of Advanced Nursing*, 25: 347–54.

Hollis, M. (1977) *Models of man*. Cambridge: Cambridge University Press.

Hopkins, C.L. (1993) Establishing a nurse-managed center: a community approach. *Nurse Practitioner Forum*, 4: 165–70.

Hunter, P. and MacAuley, D. (1996) Is this the next step for nursing? *Practice Nurse*, 23: 174–6.

Jary, D. and Jary J. (1991) *Collins dictionary of sociology*. Glasgow: Harper Collins. Jackson, C. (1995) Nurse practitioners: testing the boundaries. *Health Visitor*, 68: 135–6.

Jenkins-Clarke, S., Carr-Hill, R., Dixon, P. and Pringle, M. (1997) *Skill mix in primary care: a study of the interface between General Practitioner and other members of the primary health care team*. Executive Summary. York: Centre for Health Economics etc., The University of York.

J.M. Consulting (1999) *The regulation of nurses, midwives and health visitors: report on a review of the Nurses, Midwives and Health Visitors Act 1997*. Bristol: J.M. Consulting.

Jones, K., Gilbert, P., Little, J. *et al.* (1998) Nurse triage for house call requests in a Tyneside practice: patients' views and effect on doctor workload. *British Journal of General Practice*, 48: 1303–6.

Jordan, S. (1992) *Nurse practitioners and nurse prescribing. Learning from the US experience: a review of the literature*. Swansea: Mid West College of Nursing and Midwifery.

Kelly, G. (1981) A psychology of man himself. In: Potter, D., Anderson, J., Clarke, J. *et al.* (eds) *Society and the social sciences*. London: Routledge.

Kernick, D. (1998) Will nurses take over primary care? Talking Point. *GP Medicine*. Edn. 8, May.

Kinnersley, P., Anderson, E., Parry, K., Clement, J., Archard, L. *et al.* (2000) Randomised controlled trial of nurse practitioner versus general practitioner care for patients requesting 'same day' consultations in primary care. *British Medical Journal*, 320: 1043–8.

Knape, J. (1999) Nurses accountability in relation to nurse-led services. *British Journal of Nursing*, 8: 1514.

Kohner, N. (1994) *Clinical supervision in practice: work from nursing development units.* London: King's Fund Centre.

Lattimer, V., Sassi, F., George, S., Moore, M., Turnbull, J. *et al.* (2000) Cost analysis of nurse telephone consultation in out of hours primary care: evidence from a randomised controlled trial. *British Medical Journal*, 320: 1053–7.

Leddy, S. and Pepper J.M. (1993) *Conceptual bases of professional nursing* (third edition). Philadelphia: Lippincott.

Mackie, C. (1996) Nurse practitioners managing anticoagulant clinics. *Nursing Times*, 91: 25–8.

Marchant, C., Gupta, K., Dring, J., Shaw, S., Brewer, R. *et al.* (1997) Nurse-led pilots. *Practice Nurse*, 13: 587–91.

Marsh, G.N. and Dawes M.L. (1995) Establishing a minor-illness nurse in a busy general practice. *British Medical Journal*, 310: 778–80.

McCloskey, J.C. (1990) Two requirements for contentment: autonomy and social integration. *Journal of Nursing Scholarship*, 22: 140–3.

McGee, P., Castledine, G. and Brown, R. (1996) A survey of specialist and advanced nursing practice in England. *British Journal of Nursing*, 5: 682–6.

McGee, P. and Castledine, G. (1999) A survey of specialist and advanced nursing practice in the UK. *British Journal of Nursing*, 8: 1074–8.

McKeon, A. (1997) *Personal medical services ilots under the NHS (primary care) act 1997.* London: Stationery Office.

Medicines Control Agency (MCA). (2000) *Sale, supply and administration of medicines by health professionals under patient group directions.* Consultation Letter MLX 260. London: MCA.

Mitchinson, S. (1996) Are nurses independent and autonomous practitioners? *Nursing Standard*, 10: 34–6.

Monninger, E. (1988) A model of motivated behaviour in primary care. *Journal of Professional Nursing*, 4: 2.

Myers, P.A. (1997) Nurse practitioner is the first point of contact for urgent medical problems in a general practice setting. *Family Practice*, 14: 492–7.

NHS Executive (1998) *Personal medical services pilots under the NHS (primary care) act 1997. A comprehensive guide.* Leeds: NHS Executive.

Obeid, A. (1998) The role of the advanced practitioner in health visiting. *Journal of Community Nursing*, 12: 21–3.

Palmer, A., Burns, S. and Bulman, C. (eds) (1994) *Reflective practice in nursing: the growth of the professional practitioner.* Oxford: Blackwell Scientific Publications.

Phillips, S. (1995) Gut reaction. *Nursing Times*, 91: 44–5.

Pierce, D. and Luikart, C. (1996) Managed care: will the healthcare needs of rural citizens be met? *Journal of Nursing Administration*, 26: 28–32.

Porter, S. (1992) The poverty of professionalisation: a critical analysis of strategies for the occupational advancement of nursing. *Journal of Advanced Nursing*, 7: 720–6.

Practice Nurse. (2000) Enter high profile consultant nurses. News feature. *Practice Nurse*, 19: 49.

Proctor, S., Macey, S., Campbell, J. (1999) Clinical supervision: meeting the needs of practice nurses. *British Journal of Community Nursing*, 10: 30–9.

Read, S. (1995) *Catching the tide*. Sheffield: SCHARR, University of Sheffield.

Reverley, S. (1998) The role of the triage nurse practitioner in general medical practice: an analysis of the role. *Journal of Advanced Nursing*, 28: 584–91.

Richardson, G. and Maynard, A. (1995) *Fewer doctors? More nurses? A review of the knowledge base of doctor-nurse substitution*. Discussion paper 135. York: NHS Centre for Reviews and Dissemination, University of York.

Rogers, D.E. (1977) The challenge of primary care. In: Knowles, J.H. (ed.) *Doing better and feeling worse*. New York: W.M. Norton.

Rogers, C. (1983) *Freedom to learn for the 80s*. Columbus: Charles Merrill.

Rowley, E. (1994) The role of the practice nurse. In: Hunt, G. and Wainright, P. (eds) *Expanding the role of the nurse. The scope of professional practice*. Oxford: Blackwell Scientific.

Royal College of Nursing (RCN). (1997a) *Turning initiative into independence: information for would-be nurse entrepreneurs*. London: RCN.

Royal College of Nursing (RCN). (1997b) *Nurse practitioners: your questions answered*. London: RCN.

Ryan, S. (1997) Nurse-led monitoring in the rheumatology clinic. *Nursing Standard*, 11: 45–7.

Sackett, D., Spitzer, W., Gent. *et al.* (1974) The Burlington randomized trial of the nurse practitioner. Health outcomes of patients. *Annals of Internal Medicine*, 80: 137–42.

Salisbury, S.J. and Tettersall, M.J. 1988 Comparison of the work of a nurse practitioner with that of a general practitioner. *Journal of the Royal College of General Practitioners*, 38: 314–16.

Sams, D. (1996) Clinical supervision: an oasis for practice. *British Journal of Community Health Nursing*, 1: 87–91.

Schmidt, L., Brandt, J. and Norris, K. (1995) Nursing review. *Kansas Nurse*, 70: 1–2.

Shotter, J. (1975) *Images of man in psychological research*. London: Methuen.

Shum, C., Humphreys, A., Wheeler, D., Cochrane, M-A., Skoda, S. *et al.* (2000) Nurse management of patients with minor illnesses in general practice: multicentre, randomised controlled trial. *British Medical Journal*, 320: 1038–43.

Stevens, R. (1984) *A note on assumptions and of autonomy and determination in social psychology*. (D307 course book.) Milton Keynes: Open University Press.

Stein, L.M. (1993) Health delivery to farm workers in the southwest: an innovative nursing clinic. *Journal of the American Academic Nurse Practitioners*, 5: 119–24.

Stilwell, B., Greenfield S., Dinny, M. *et al.* (1987) A nurse practitioner in general practice: working styles and pattern of consultations. *Journal of the Royal College of General Practitioners*, 37: 154–7.

Styles, J., Casey, C. and Gibson, T. (1999) Is clinical supervision an option for practice nurses? *Practice Nursing*, 10: 11.

Sultz, H. (1983) *A study of nurse practitioner programs*. Washington DC: National Technical Information Service.

Tingle, J. (1997) Expanded role of the nurse: accountability confusion. *British Journal of Nursing*, 6: 1011–13.

Torn, A. and McNichol, E. (1996) Can a mental health nurse be a nurse practitioner? *Nursing Standard*, 11: 39–44.

Tortora, G.J. and Grabowski, S.R. (1996) *Principles of anatomy and physiology* (eighth edition). New York: Harper Collins.

Touche Ross. (1996) *Evaluation of nurse practitioner pilot projects: final report.* London: NHS Executive South Thames.

Twinn, S., Roberts, B. and Andrews, S. (1996) *Community health care nursing principles for practice.* Oxford: Butterworth Heineman.

United Kingdom Central Council (UKCC). (1992a) *Code of professional conduct for the nurse, midwife and health visitor.* London: UKCC.

United Kingdom Central Council (UKCC). (1992b) The scope of professional practice. London: UKCC.

United Kingdom Central Council (UKCC). (1994) *The future of professional practice – the Council's standards for education and practice following registration.* London: UKCC.

United Kingdom Central Council (UKCC). (1996a) *Guidelines for professional practice.* London: UKCC.

United Kingdom Central Council (UKCC). (1996b) *PREP – the nature of advanced practice – an interim report.* CC/96/46. London: UKCC.

United Kingdom Central Council (UKCC). (1997a) *PREP – the nature of advanced practice.* London: UKCC.

United Kingdom Central Council (UKCC). (1997b) *PREP – specialist practice. Consideration of issues relating to embracing nurse practitioners and clinical nurse specialists within the specialist practice framework.* London: UKCC.

United Kingdom Central Council (UKCC). (1998) *A higher level of practice: consultation document.* London: UKCC.

United Kingdom Central Council (UKCC). (1999a) *A higher level of practice: report of the consultation on the UKCC's proposals for a revised regulatory framework for post-registration clinical practice.* London: UKCC.

United Kingdom Central Council (UKCC). (1999b) *A higher level of practice: draft descriptor and standard – testing and validation.* London: UKCC.

United Kingdom Central Council (UKCC). (1999c) *Register.* 28. London: UKCC.

United Kingdom Central Council (UKCC). (1999d) *A higher level of practice pilot.* London: UKCC.

United Kingdom Central Council (UKCC). (1999e) *The continuing professional development standard: information for registered nurses, midwives and health visitors.* London: UKCC.

United Kingdom Central Council (UKCC). (2000) *Register.* 30. London: UKCC.

United Kingdom Central Council (UKCC). (2000b). *The practice standard information for registered nurses, midwives and health vistors.* London: UKCC.

Venning, P., Durie, A., Roland, M., Roberts, C. and Leese, B. (2000) Randomised controlled trial comparing cost effectiveness of general practitioners and nurse practitioners in primary care. *British Medical Journal,* 320: 1048–53.

Vrabec, N. (1995) Implications of US healthcare reform for the rural elderly. *Nursing Outlook,* 43: 260–5.

While, A. (1999) The new Council: will it provide the basis for a sound profession? *British Journal of Community Nursing,* 4: 137–8.

Wilkinson, J. (1997) Developing a concept analysis of autonomy in nursing practice. *British Journal of Nursing,* 6: 703–7.

Williams, A. and Sibbald, B. (1999) Changing roles and identities in primary health care: exploring a culture of uncertainty. *Journal of Advanced Nursing,* 29: 737–45.

Whitehouse, C. (1994) A new source of support: the nurse practitioner role in Parkinson's disease and dystonia. *Professional Nurse,* 9: 450–1.

Woodman, J. (1997) Nurse triage: easing the workload. *Practice Nurse,* 14: 554–8.

Ethical and legal considerations of community nursing

Marc A. Cornock

Introduction

Ethical and legal considerations of nursing are not purely academic; they have consequences for the way in which individual practitioners think about and perform their roles. Community nurses may be seen as independent practitioners in the true sense of the term; often, they are isolated from their colleagues when performing their professional duties. Recent initiatives have reinforced the call for more interprofessional and multi-agency working. In order for this to be effective, the members of the team need to be clear about their roles and the boundaries within which they are working.

This chapter will not address the legal framework for providing community care in the UK, such as the National Health Service and Community Care Act 1990. Rather, it will examine and discuss the ethics and law concerning nursing practice in the community setting. Also, how the nurse, working in this setting, is affected by ethical and legal considerations.

Primary health care has been undergoing continuous change in recent years. Although this change continues, the ethical and legal principles, which affect nursing practice, remain the same. For instance, nurse prescribing is a recent addition to the role of the community nurse; however, in performing this role nurses have to observe the same duty of care to their clients as they have always done.

It is important to note that the method of citing legal cases can be confusing to the uninitiated. Therefore references will be supplied to textbooks that discuss relevant cases rather than to the original cases themselves.

Ethical and legal framework

Nurses do not work in a vacuum but in a society. It is therefore logical to assume that they will be working according to the norms and values of that society. However, the individuals that comprise society will have differing views on what is and is not important to them, and the value that they apply to these views. For instance, respect is a value that many people hold dear and apply in their daily lives. Yet there are other members of our society who, it may be said, have little respect for others in the way they live their lives.

It is our personal values, beliefs and attitudes that inform our ethical stance and also, our professional practice as nurses. When there is a decision to be made, it is our values and beliefs that aid this process.

It may be said that there are two major approaches to ethical or moral decision-making, the 'deontological' or 'teleological'. The former sees everyone as being equal and actions as being good or bad in their own right; thus, there should be equality in the treatment of individuals. This approach has been forwarded by those such as Immanuel Kant (1973). The other approach, put forward by those such as John Stuart Mill and Jeremy Bentham (Beauchamp and Childress, 1994), sees actions in terms of their consequence. It is commonly termed the 'greatest happiness principle', as it is based upon happiness or pleasure as determinants of the greatest outcome for the greatest number of people.

Ethics are merely a framework upon which we base our nursing practice. It defines some of the values and beliefs of the profession. We cannot break an ethical principle in the same way that a law can be broken. Rather, we choose to uphold the principle or not, depending upon whether we agree with it or not. The law, on the other hand, does not give us the same option of choice. However, ethics and law are interrelated; ethics may be influenced by what is legal and the law is influenced by ethics.

It is simplest to think of the law as a set of rules adopted by society. These rules are enforceable by a legal system that includes the police service and the courts. The purpose of the legal system is to ensure that the rules are followed and that anyone who does not follow the rules is punished. This act of punishment becomes a deterrent to others who are considering breaking the rules of society.

Reference to the British legal system, in fact, refers to the common legal system that exists in England and Wales. Northern Ireland and Scotland have their own separate and distinct legal systems.

There are two main areas to the legal system of England and Wales: criminal and civil. The criminal system is concerned with punishment of wrongdoers and is initiated by the state, with the intention of preventing anti-social behaviour. The civil system, on the other hand, is concerned with actions brought by one individual or organization against another, its intent being to regulate the interactions between individuals and organizations.

Foundation of law in England and Wales

England and Wales has two main forms of law, which are evolved through Statute and Common law. Parliament exercises its law-making ability given to it by society through Acts of Parliament, normally known as 'Statutes'. For an Act of Parliament to be received into law it needs to pass through both Houses of Parliament and receive the Royal Assent.

When the courts cannot turn to a relevant statute, because there is no particular Act of Parliament that regulates that specific area of law, they turn to Common law. Common law is sometimes referred to as 'case law', or 'precedent'. It refers to the practice of looking to previous examples, or cases, to see what has been decided or, how statutes have been interpreted in a particular case to see if they have a bearing on the particular case before the court. The justice system of England and Wales has tiers of courts. A lower court is bound by a decision of a higher court, that is it has to apply the principles of law enshrined in a higher court if it has a bearing on the case before them, a system known as precedent.

European law is having increasing influence on the law of England and Wales. When the UK signed the Treaty of Rome, in 1973, it meant that the laws and regulations passed by the European Community (EC) would have effect in British law.

An example of Statute is that of the United Kingdom Central Council for Nurses, Midwives and Health Visitors (UKCC), which was set up as a result of the Nurses, Midwives and Health Visitors Act of 1979. Medical negligence law, however, has developed through the common law system, using precedent to establish its principles.

PROFESSIONAL FRAMEWORK

As stated, the regulation of nursing is enshrined in an Act of Parliament, the Nurses, Midwives and Health Visitors Act 1979. The Act is responsible for the creation of the UKCC and the four National Boards of England, Northern Ireland, Scotland and Wales.

The primary purpose of the UKCC is the protection of the public from nurses unfit to practice, whether they are trained, untrained or bogus. Everyone who wishes to practise as a nurse in the UK is required to register with the UKCC. If an individual is not on the register he or she cannot work as a qualified nurse in the UK. Thus, any nurse who was struck off the register would be unable to practise his or her profession. Complaints of misconduct are heard by the professional conduct committee of the UKCC.

Circulars and advisory documents issued by the UKCC or the government do not have the force of law behind them, but instead are to be taken as accepted practice in courts of law. For instance, the UKCC code of conduct sets out the accepted conduct of a nurse. However, a nurse would not be liable in a court of law for merely not following the code. It is important to note though, that deviance from the code may be seen as evidence of falling below the standard required of a professional nurse or of misconduct on the part of the nurse. Thus failing to follow the code could be used against the nurse as evidence of a poor standard of care.

PROFESSIONAL CODE OF CONDUCT

The UKCC has issued a code of professional conduct (UKCC, 1992a), designed to assist nurses in deciding upon what is the appropriate conduct in any situation. The original code of professional conduct was issued in 1984 and the current version, issued in 1992, is the third edition.

Codes of conduct are based upon ethical and legal principles and change as these principles change. Thus codes of conduct are not static documents but evolve over time to suit the society that they serve. They do not provide definitive answers to the professionals they cover but guide their practice.

EXTENSION OF ROLES AND PROFESSIONAL PRACTICE

There has been, and still is, much discussion within nursing as to what constitutes a nursing duty and what constitutes a non-nursing duty. Until relatively recently, 1992, there existed within nursing the concept of extended roles. Nursing duties were what was taught during nurse training, with a syllabus prescribed by the General Nursing Council. Any other duty was non-nursing. However, over time, more and more duties and functions were added to the nurse's role. Those that were not incorporated into basic, or pre-registration, training were termed extended roles. For nurses to undertake these additional roles they had to receive additional training that was recognized by their employing health authority as satisfactory for the purpose. Additionally, nurses had to adhere to policies and procedures concerning the additional role, that were issued by the health authority.

There has been a move away from extended roles in recent years and, with the publication of *Scope of Professional Practice* (UKCC, 1992b), the concept has been superseded by the notion of professional competence. For the UKCC, professional competence means that nurses are not limited in their professional practice. Rather, nurses are free to undertake any duty for which they have the necessary skill, knowledge and competence. There are several principles that nurses have to adhere to within the *Scope of Professional Practice* (UKCC, 1992b), such as always acting in the interests of the patient; acknowledging their own limitations; keeping themselves up to date regarding their skills, knowledge and competence; not compromising standards by undertaking advanced roles, and recognizing their own accountability.

Whilst this development may be seen as an advancement in nursing skills and competencies, it may place nurses in a dilemma as to whether they actually possess the relevant skills, knowledge and competence to undertake the role. For nurses working in isolation from their colleagues, as in the community, this may be particularly problematic. The UKCC has put the accountability for accepting roles firmly on the nurse who accepts them. Nurses taking on additional roles and duties, prescribing for instance, should ensure that they are competent to do so. With nurse prescribing there is a recognized educational course that community nurses have to attend before being able to prescribe for their clients. However, for many roles there is no such course and nurses may be left unsure as to whether they are actually competent. Where nurses have cause to doubt their competence to undertake a role or task, they should not assume responsibility or accountability for it but request the assistance of another colleague or health care professional.

Having outlined the ethical and legal framework within which community nurses work, the following sections discuss various ethical and legal problems that nurses working in community settings may encounter.

PATIENTS' RIGHTS

Although there is no absolute right to receive community care in the UK, all patients have certain rights in their dealings with health care professionals. In 1995 the government issued *The Patient's Charter* (DOH, 1995) to inform patients of some of their rights. The rights contained within the charter are not all legally enforceable, as only some of the 'rights' were pre-existing rights which are legally enforceable. An example of a pre-existing right, that is legally enforceable, is access to health care records (this will be discussed later).

CONFIDENTIALITY

It is generally accepted that health care practitioners owe a duty of confidence to their patients, in respect of information they acquire in their capacity as health care practitioners. This duty of confidence is a legal obligation that arises as part of a contract, whether implied or explicit, by virtue of a general legal duty, and as part of Common law. It may be said that confidentiality is one of the most fundamental ethical obligations owed by health care practitioners to their patients. Respect of the confidences of the patient is enshrined in the Hippocratic oath and the Declaration of Geneva, and repeated in professional codes of conduct such as that issued by the UKCC (1992a). The basis of the principle of confidentiality is that patients are able to fully disclose all their symptoms and problems and so aid diagnosis and treatment, because health care practitioners will keep all information divulged to them, or discovered by them in examination, secret.

For a discussion on confidentiality and the nurse see clause 10 of the *Code of Professional Conduct* (UKCC, 1992a), which makes reference to confidential information. This clause has been expanded upon by the UKCC, see *Guidelines for Professional Practice* (UKCC, 1996). However, the clause does not discuss what actually constitutes confidential information. Is information confidential merely because a patient has entrusted you with it, or must it have some specific quality about it? For instance, as a community nurse, would a client informing you that he or she was unemployed count as confidential information?

The law surrounding breach of confidence has arisen in the first instance from case law. This has resulted in various principles that have been re-applied and expanded upon in various cases since they were first delivered. The various principles concerning confidentiality and breach of confidence include that: the information must be something that has the necessary quality of confidence (saying that one had a motor car would not count as confidential information as it would be possible for others to know this fairly easily); the information must not already be in the public domain, that is, it is not something that is already known; the information must have been imparted in circumstances that imply an obligation of confidence. The nurse's *Code of Professional Conduct* (UKCC, 1992a) makes it quite clear that information received in the course of one's duty would fulfil this third criterion, although general impersonal information is unlikely to be seen as confidential. Also, information obtained through case conferences or patients' notes is afforded the same degree of confidentiality, as if patients had passed on the information themselves.

Finally, it must be in the public interest to protect the information. This means that not all information will be subject to the duty of confidentiality and that this duty is not absolute, meaning that there are circumstances when the confidence can be legally breached. For instance, if it is in the public interest for the information to be disclosed then the health care practitioner can disclose it, for example certain communicable diseases, or homicidal intention towards a specific person could be disclosed. Thus the example given above, of a patient disclosing that he or she was unemployed, would not count as confidential if it was widely known that this was so.

The best advice that can be given to nurses is that any information that they come into contact with through their duties should be regarded as being confidential. It is important to note that if harm were to occur to a patient as a result of a breach of confidentiality, it could amount to a form of negligence because it would constitute a breach of the standard of care required. The general principles stated above apply to all information received by health care practitioners about patients in the course of their professional work.

It is worth noting that disclosure of information to a health care professional, even a confession, is not privileged. In fact, the only privilege with regard to confidentiality and privileged information is between clients and their lawyers. Everyone else, even a priest, can be sent to prison if they refuse to give evidence or divulge information when directed to do so by a court.

It was noted above that the obligation of confidence is not absolute. Disclosure of so-called confidential information can be required by the courts, in the public interest and by statute. There are a number of statutory provisions that create exceptions to the rule of confidentiality, for example the Police and Criminal Evidence Act 1984, Abortion Regulations 1991.

With regard to the disclosure of confidential information in the public interest, it is important to note that it must be in the public interest and not because the public would be interested in the information. It is generally accepted that the public interest criterion is satisfied when failure to disclose information may expose the patient or others to death or risk of serious harm. This may occur with a patient driving against medical advice; there is a public interest in informing the Driver and Vehicle Licensing Authority (DVLA). Similarly, if a colleague is putting patients at risk as a result of illness, there would be a public interest in informing the employer or UKCC. The detection and prevention of serious crime is also a public interest exception to the principle of confidentiality.

However, it has also been established that there is a public interest in loyalty, mutual trust and confidentiality between patients and their health care practitioners. Other public interests must be weighed against this public interest and against private rights. Also, any disclosure may be made in the public interest but must be made to the relevant authority and not to just anyone.

Of course, any information may be disclosed with the express consent of the patient. Thus, if there is information that needs to be shared with others, it is advisable to ask patients to give their consent. If this consent is not forthcoming, the information may only be divulged if the disclosure can be said to fall into one of the categories discussed above.

For nurses and other health professionals working as part of a team, it is important that information is freely transferable between the relevant team members in order for patients to receive effective care and treatment. Therefore, it is assumed that patients consent to this transfer of information unless they explicitly forbid it.

Confidential information is also needed for the purposes of research, auditing and teaching. In these circumstances patients should be approached for their consent. Where this is not possible any details obtained should be anonymised so that patients cannot be identified. Patients should be told that information they provide may be passed to others, and that they are entitled to withhold their consent.

There are always times when information needs to be passed to a third person or agency quickly, when there is not time to undertake administrative procedures to gain permission to pass on the information and consent is not forthcoming from the provider of the information. As a general rule, in exceptional circumstances, it is permissible to disclose information to a third party, such as a close relative or appropriate authority (e.g. social worker). However, this has to be undertaken in the best interests of patients, for example if the patient is a child and suspected of being abused.

PATIENT RECORDS

Patient records are an important aspect of a patients' care and treatment. The records should always be treated as confidential; if they are used for purposes other than determining patients' treatment, this could constitute a breach of confidence.

If there is any complaint or question over the care or treatment that a patient received it will be the records that are looked to for evidence. Well-written, comprehensive records can often prove to be the health care professional's greatest ally in defending allegations of breach of duty of care. It is important that records are legible, written in a common language, comprehensive and concise. All entries must be signed by the person making the entry and have the date and time entered. It is not unknown for patient records to be used in a court some considerable time after they were made; therefore, the notes need to be meaningful to the person making them.

Where records are left in patients' homes, there is a tendency for less information to be recorded. This is perfectly acceptable provided that the record contains the necessary information for any other health care professional to continue with the care and treatment. Any additional information could be kept at the nurse's office or base, with a note on the record stating that there is additional information available.

There are various statutes that deal with a patient's rights in relation to access to health records, including the Data Protection Act 1984 and Access to Health Records Act 1990. Together, these Acts cover access to automated and manual records. Essentially, patients have the right to apply for access to the records held about them. However, there is no automatic right for patients to receive access and access can be denied for any record made before the date of the Act. It is the record holder who makes the decision regarding access. Access may be withheld, for instance, if the information identifies another person who has supplied information about the patient, though if this individual consents access can be allowed. Also, if the information in the record is likely to cause serious physical or mental harm to the health of the patient, access may be denied. If the decision is made that part of the record would cause serious harm to the patient's health, there are two options: to refuse access to the record as a whole or to allow limited access to the record, excluding that part which is deemed to be harmful to the patient.

Once patients have access to their records they can challenge the accuracy of the information they contain and ask for corrections to be made to any inaccurate information.

It was stated above that additional notes may be kept on patients in addition to any that are left with them. If this is the case any additional notes may have an application for access made on them. When a request for access is made it is for the full record, subject to the possibility of harm to the patient.

Consent to treatment

The basic principle of consent may be said to have been laid down by Justice Cardozo as long ago as 1914 in an American case. He stated that:

> Every human being of adult years and sound mind has a right to determine what shall be done with his own body; and a surgeon who performs an operation without his patient's consent commits an assault . . . (J. Cardozo in *Schloendorff v. Society of New York Hospital 1914* (Kennedy and Grubb, 1994: 87)

All nurses must be aware that any treatment needs the patient's consent before the treatment can begin. It is unlawful to touch another person without their consent (see trespass to person below).

Many people believe that obtaining consent is related to obtaining a signature on a consent form. This is certainly not the legal position on consent. It is considered good practice to have consent forms that require the patient's signature, although consent does not have to be written, it can be given verbally or even implied. However, when they are used, consent forms should not be seen as a form of 'blank cheque' that allows health care professionals to undertake whatever procedure they wish. Consent forms should be used to demonstrate the patient has consented to specific identified procedures, except in exceptional circumstances (see below). Practice nurses who undertake 'flu immunizations would not necessarily need to obtain written consent from each patent, providing that the patient consents verbally or by inference (see below).

INFORMED CONSENT

Obtaining a signature on a consent form does not fulfil the legal requirements for obtaining a patient's consent to a procedure. The principle of informed consent, 'the duty of completely disclosing information to a patient as to medical treatment before it is undertaken' (Curzon, 1996) is not enforced by British law; this was established in the case of *Sidaway v. Bethlem Royal Hospital Governors 1984* (see Kennedy and Grubb, 1994: 152). This case involved a woman who consented to an operation, suffered damaged to her spinal cord and sued because she said that the surgeon did not warn her of the risk of this occurring. The judges in the case were of the opinion that the surgeon did not have to inform her of all the possible risks involved with the operation.

The law merely states that patients need to receive information that allows them to make an informed decision to give or withhold consent. For instance, with regard to an operation, patients may be informed of why the operation is necessary, what the operation entails, and any inherent risk, although what constitutes a risk is a matter that, in the British courts, is usually decided via medical paternalism. It is up to the health care practitioners to decide upon the nature and scope of information that they give to their patients. However, the health care practitioner could be sued, in a civil court under the tort of negligence (see below), if patients do not believe that they were given reasonable information and that the practitioner was failing in his or her duty of care. Thus, best practice is to give full information whenever possible.

All information that is given to patients must be given in a language that they will understand. Any decision to withhold information from patients must be justified. If there is a decision not to provide full information to a patient, a very careful assessment of the degree of harm, that may be caused to the patient by providing full information, must be made. Note that consent obtained through coercion or undue influence ('improper pressure on a person resulting in his being at a manifest disadvantage' (Curzon, 1996)) is invalid.

CONSENT BY OTHERS

Once a person has reached the age of 18, the only person who can give consent on their behalf is the person himself or herself. This principle applies whether the patient is competent or incompetent. There is no legal validity to consent being obtained from the relatives of an adult.

Thus the unconscious patient, or the person who is incompetent because of a lack of understanding, is incapable of giving consent on his or her own behalf, and it is not possible for anyone to give consent on his or her behalf. This situation is not as bizarre as it may first appear. The purpose of this principle of being unable to consent on behalf of another is to protect individuals. It does not mean that they cannot receive treatment or care.

Instead, if a person is incompetent or incapable of giving consent, for whatever reason, medical treatment can be justified on the doctrine of necessity, unless it conflicts with the known wishes of the patient. When dealing with a client who cannot give consent, the best course of action is always to act in the best interests of the client. This means that the practitioner has to consider whether the client needs the procedure or treatment and, if there is a possibility of side-effects for the client, whether the risks outweigh the benefits to the client. It is usually the people who will be performing the procedure that have to convince themselves that the proposed treatment is in the client's best interests. The procedure to be followed would be to decide that the treatment is warranted in the client's best interests, and to treat the client without asking for consent from anyone.

However, the doctrine of necessity may only be invoked if the treatment is necessary either to save the client's life or to ensure improvement, or prevent deterioration, in their physical or mental well-being. Only treatment that is necessary for the above reasons should be undertaken under the doctrine of necessity.

This principle applies to therapeutic treatments, such as practice nurses treating a collapsed patient, community nurses treating a client with diabetes who is hyperglycaemic. However, if non-therapeutic treatment (e.g. sterilization) is being considered for a client who is incapable of consenting (for example, a client with learning disability), this normally requires the approval of the courts, who will decide upon their interpretation of the best interests of the individual.

In the situation where the patient has consented to an operation but during the surgery it is discovered that an additional procedure is warranted, the surgeon may act in order to save the patient's life or to preserve the health of the patient. In all other cases, the patient should be allowed to recover and then consent obtained for the additional surgery.

CONSENT FOR A CHILD/MINOR

A minor, for purposes of consent, is someone under the age of 16. Once minors reach the age of 16, their consent is as valid as an adult's. Before minors can give consent for a procedure they need to have their competence to give that consent assessed. This means that they need to have sufficient understanding and intelligence (known as 'Gillick competence') to enable them to fully understand what is being proposed (Montgomery, 1997: 284). However, it is worth noting that even if a person under 16 has the necessary understanding and intelligence, it does not prevent the necessary consent being obtained from another competent source, for example, the parents (Montgomery, 1997: 285).

If a minor, deemed as being Gillick competent, consents to a proposed treatment, the parents cannot veto the treatment. However, if the parents consent on the minor's behalf, the minor cannot veto their consent. Whilst this may seem unjust, woolly, and apparently against the Children Act 1989, the principle has been upheld by the Court of Appeal. However, courts have the power to override the consent of the parents where it is deemed not to be in the best interests of the child.

It may be useful to think of consent and the child as a lock and key, with the consent being the key. All health professional need is one key to turn the lock, this can come from the parents, the child, the courts or even health professional themselves if they are acting in an emergency and in the child's best interests. For instance, a school nurse giving a child an immunization would undertake resuscitation measures if the child developed anaphylaxis.

INFERRED CONSENT

Although consent has to be given for any procedure, as stated above, this does not have to be in writing, nor does it have to be given verbally. There is also the principle of inferred consent. Kennedy and Grubb (1998) note that inferred consent refers to the situation where:

> . . . a patient who allows a doctor to carry out a procedure in full knowledge of what is to be done will have given actual consent to the procedure. . . . The fact that the patient did not express his consent is not conclusive. Rather, faced with these facts, what other inference is it proper for the court to make other than the patient was actually consenting'
>
> (Kennedy and Grubb, 1998:125–6).

The classical example of inferred consent is the individual who joins a queue of people receiving immunizations, who is told that he or she will receive an immunization, they roll up their sleeve when asked to do so, proffer an arm and receive the injection. Although the individual does not sign a consent form or give verbal consent, consent is inferred from the actions he or she takes.

TRESPASS TO PERSON

If legal consent has not been given for a procedure then trespass to the person is said to have occurred. This will usually be one of two forms, assault or battery. There is some confusion about what these two terms mean. *Assault* is said to occur when a person is put in fear of 'unlawful physical violence' (Curzon, 1996), whereas *battery* is the 'direct use of unlawful force on a person without his consent' (Curzon, 1996). Thus, assault is the fear of violence whilst battery is the actual execution of that threat.

Terminal care

This is an area that can pose considerable dilemmas for health care professionals. It is not unlawful to withhold a diagnosis from a dying patient, as patients do not have an automatic right to full information regarding their condition and diagnosis, under British law. However, although accepted practice, if the health care professional decides to withhold information from the patient only to subsequently inform the relatives there could be a breach of confidentiality, with the result that the patient may sue the community nurse.

Euthanasia, as in bringing about the death of someone suffering from an incurable illness or disease, is illegal in the UK. This is regardless of whether one believes it to be a mercy killing, active euthanasia, passive euthanasia, assisting suicide or voluntary euthanasia. Regardless of the terminology, intentionally causing the death of another will result in a homicide charge. However, all health care professionals wish a peaceful death for their patients when there is no further treatment that can be given.

The law is quite specific about what is and is not permissible. Whilst the taking of one's own life is not a criminal offence, assisting another to do so is a criminal offence. It is recognized by the law that there are times when it is inevitable that the patient is going to die. It is accepted that the relief of suffering is a fundamental aspect of a health professional's role. This is acknowledged in what has come to be known as the 'doctrine of double effect'. This was first established in the case of *R v. Bodkin-Adams*. In this case, concerning a doctor being charged with murder, Mr Justice Devlin stated:

> ... if the first purpose of medicine, the restoration of health, can no longer be achieved, there is still much for the doctor to do, and he is entitled to do all that is proper and necessary to relieve pain and suffering, even if the measures he takes may incidentally shorten life.
>
> (Kennedy and Grubb, 1998: 271)

This refers to the situation where a patient with a terminal illness is receiving morphine to relieve his or her pain and suffering. There will come a point when the dosage of morphine they receive may shorten their life. What the doctrine of double effect means in practice is, that if the intention of the person providing a dose of morphine is to relieve the patient's suffering, then there is a lawful reason for the action and the health care professional would not be held to have committed murder or manslaughter. The incidental death of the patient, although anticipated, is not the desired outcome.

Any competent patient may refuse treatment, even if that refusal will result in their death. Also, treatment may be withdrawn or withheld from patients, if it is in their best interests to do so. The law recognizes that it is not always appropriate for a patient to receive active treatment, especially when that treatment has no therapeutic purpose.

Advance directives, sometimes referred to as 'living wills', where individuals decide against medical treatment in anticipation of their needing it at some point in the future, often pose problems for health care professionals. There is uncertainty as to their validity, which has not been tested in the courts of England and Wales, although some commentators are of the opinion that the judges in the case of *Airedale NHS Trust v. Bland* confirmed their legal effect (Kennedy and Grubb 1994: 1327). At present, best practice would be to obtain legal advice from health care trust solicitors.

Accountability and professional liability

Part of being a professional is being accountable for one's actions. Accountability is different to responsibility because it is possible to be responsible for one's actions without being held to account for them. Accountability suggests that the practitioner is acting with authority and has the autonomy to decide which course of action to take, or even whether to act at all. It is not something that can be assumed at one moment and then left at another. As professionals, community nurses are accountable for their actions at all times. Accountability means being able to justify and explain and defend actions. However, accountability is not just concerned with being able to account for one's actions, it also means being able to justify one's omissions.

There may be said to be four spheres in which nurses are accountable. There is the moral accountability that nurses owe to themselves, justifying one's actions to oneself. Then there is the accountability nurses owe to their employers, justifying their actions in terms of their role in the organization. All nurses, as members of a professional register, are accountable to their fellow nurses and the profession as a whole, for instance undertaking practice in accordance with the code of professional practice. Finally, there is legal accountability, the duty of care that exists between nurses and their patients.

If a nurse is guilty of professional misconduct, even where there is no harm caused to the patient, he or she may have to face a disciplinary hearing of the professional conduct committee of the UKCC. The central issue will be whether the nurse has followed the UKCC *Code of Professional Conduct* (UKCC, 1992a) and any further guidelines laid down by the UKCC or English National Board for Nursing, Midwifery and Health Visiting (ENB).

PROFESSIONAL NEGLIGENCE

It is often said that patients are becoming more and more litigious. They are willing to use the courts to exercise what they see as their rights. National Health Service patients do not have a contract with the health care professionals who treat them, and so they are not able to bring legal actions in contract law. Rather, most malpractice cases are heard under the tort of negligence.

However, as stated above, professional nurses are accountable for their actions and legally liable for any malpractice they perform. In the legal sense, liability means a legal obligation or duty. Patients have a right to expect certain standards of care, and if the care falls below this standard they have a right to seek redress. Thus the nurse caring for a patient has a liability to do so in a safe and competent manner. If the liability is not upheld, the nurse may be accused of acting negligently. This negligence could give rise to a criminal prosecution, if it was in the form of a criminal act, e.g. assaulting a patient, or a civil suit if the patient decided to sue (to sue someone means to take legal proceedings against them).

Many health care professionals feel that the law is weighted against them if a patient decides to sue them for negligence. Whilst it is undoubtedly true that defending a negligence case is an unpleasant experience, the burden of proof falls almost entirely onto the patient and the standard of proof is set by the profession itself.

The patient who has suffered harm, or the person acting on his or her behalf, must establish the following facts:

- That a duty of care was owed to him/her by the defendant (the community nurse).
- That this duty was breached.
- That the outcome was caused by the breach of duty (known as causation) and was reasonably foreseeable.
- That harm resulted.

Duty of care

In order to win his or her case the plaintiff [patient] must show that a duty of care was owed to them by the defendant [community nurse]. Usually it is relatively easy for the plaintiff to establish that a duty of care was owed to them. A duty arises as a matter of law where a professional is caring for a client, undertaking tasks as part of their normal and recognized duties. Thus, professionals all have a duty of care to their patients and clients.

Breach of the duty of care

Before it can be established whether there has been a breach of the duty of care, it is necessary to determine the standard of care expected of the professional in the particular set of circumstances.

In *Bolam v. Friern Hospital Management Committee 1957* (Kennedy and Grubb, 1994), Mr Justice McNair defined the standard of care as:

> The standard of the ordinary skilled man exercising and professing to have that special skill . . . In the case of a medical man negligence means failure to act in accordance with the standards of reasonably competent medical men at the time. But it must be remembered that there may be one or more perfectly proper standards; and if a medical man conforms with one of those proper standards then he is not negligent.
>
> (Kennedy and Grubb, 1994: 441)

Although this case was specifically about doctors, the so-called medical man, it has since been applied to all health care professionals, including community specialist practitioners who work autonomously and often in isolation. It is not sufficient for the plaintiff to establish that there is a body of competent professional opinion that considers your decision wrong, if there is also a body of equally competent professional opinion that supports your decision. This is basically saying that the law imposes a duty of care; but the standard of care is a matter of professional judgement. Thus, a community nurse would be judged against another community nurse of similar experience and qualification to gauge the acceptable standard of care.

For nurses, the standard of care will encompass the UKCC *Code of Professional Conduct* (UKCC, 1992a) and any standards that the UKCC and other processional bodies have drawn up, e.g. *Scope of Professional Practice* (UKCC, 1992b). The specialist practitioner must demonstrate a greater standard of care and therefore greater skill in undertaking the task than an unqualified individual.

In today's health culture with its emphasis on policies, protocols and evidence-based practice, failing to follow such protocols will need to be carefully explained by the practitioner in order to demonstrate that the duty of care was not breached.

Causation

Having established that there was a duty of care owed to the patient and that this duty was breached, the plaintiff has to demonstrate that it was the breach in the duty that caused reasonably foreseeable harm to the patient. It is on this establishment of a causal link that most negligence cases are either won or lost.

Harm

The final element that the plaintiff has to establish is that harm was suffered as a result of the breach. Actions for negligence will inevitably fail if there has been no harm suffered. The definition of harm includes loss or damage of property as well as personal injury or death, for example, inappropriate treatment of a client with a leg ulcer, causing the patient harm either from the treatment itself or because the leg ulcer takes longer to heal.

VICARIOUS LIABILITY

Employers are vicariously liable for the actions of their employees acting in the course of their employment. In practice this means that the employer will be the one who will be sued, not the individual nurse, and that the employer will provide legal support for the employee.

All employees are covered by the concept of vicarious liability when working within the normal confines of their role; therefore nurses would have to prove that they were employees acting in the course of their employment. It is relatively easy to prove one is an employee; in most instances this merely involves providing a contract of employment. The more difficult aspect is proving that you are acting in the course of your employment, although job descriptions and accepted working practices are sometimes helpful here. The continuing changing aspect of community nursing means that job descriptions are not always relevant to what the community nurse actually undertakes. As the role evolves the job description does not always evolve alongside.

Nurses' rights in relation to patients

When considering the ethical and legal principles affecting nurses working in community settings, one should remember that the principles are there to protect the nurse as well as the patient (see occupiers liability below).

OCCUPIERS' LIABILITY

The liability of occupiers to visitors entering their premises is enshrined in legislation, Occupiers' Liability Act 1957. The purpose of the Act is to protect visitors from suffering injury as a direct result of being in or on the property. The occupier is regarded as the person in control or possession of the property, whereas a visitor is anyone who has been invited, by the occupier, on to the premises. Thus, the occupier has a duty to all visitors to ensure that they will be reasonably safe whilst using the premises. If an accident were to befall the nurse working in a patient's home, there could be a case for action against the patient, if the accident were as a result of negligence.

Of note is the fact that the Act only places a duty on the occupier in relation to a visitor to the premises. The provisions of the Act do not cover anyone who is not invited on to the property. Thus, if the nurse were asked to leave and refused to do so, they would not receive the cover of the Act if they were to hurt themselves. Another point of note is that the Act only covers the visitor for the purpose for which they are invited into the property. If, whilst there, the nurse undertakes anything outside of his or her nursing duties, they would not receive the same cover under the Act.

For those persons who are not deemed visitors (i.e. trespassers), the Occupiers' Liability Act 1984 provides limited protection against suffering harm as a result of being on the property.

It is unlikely that a nurse would be a trespasser in a patient's home and so would receive the protection of the Occupiers' Liability Act 1957, rather than the 1984 Act. However, the difference in protection between the two Acts means that it is important for nurses to ensure that they are entering the right address, that they are invited to enter, and that when asked to do so, they leave.

The occupier always has a right to ask a visitor to leave and could use reasonable force to comply a visitor to do so. Nurses have no authority, as a result of their profession, that absolves them from committing trespass when asked to leave.

GIFTS

It is common for patients to present gifts to nurses. Many nurses feel that acceptance of these gifts places them in a difficult ethical and legal position. There is no legal contraindication to receiving a gift from a patient, no law that states nurses should not accept gifts of gratitude. The legal difficulty for community nurses would be in proving that an item was a gift given to them and not something that they had removed from the patient's house.

Ethically, there are dilemmas in accepting gifts from patients. Most patients give gifts as an expression of their gratitude to a nurse. It is a genuine gift and represents a 'thank you' to the nurse from the patient. However, nurses must be aware of the patient who is trying to use the gift to gain undue influence over the nurse or favours from them in return. There are also patients from whom it may be inappropriate to receive a gift, for instance, those with dementia or conditions that affect their judgement. Some patients may feel obliged to present a gift to a nurse who has been working in their home for a considerable time, they may come to see the nurse as an extension of their family and friends, whilst others, who feel dependent upon the nurse, may give a gift in an attempt to maintain a relationship.

It can be very difficult to refuse a gift from a patient. However, a nurse being offered a gift has to give careful consideration before accepting it. Any local policies on the receipt of gifts will have to be adhered to and it is useful to find these out before a gift is offered.

Where the nurse is unsure as to whether to accept a gift, but has accepted it to prevent offence or because of the insistence of the patient, discussing the matter with managers and other colleagues may help to clarify the dilemma. In general, gifts of small or negligible value, such as chocolates or something made by the patient, can be accepted, as can gifts at the end of a treatment, where the nurse is not expecting to come into contact with that patient again. Nurses usually get to know their patients fairly well and can assess the situation in which the gift is being given. If the nurse feels wary of accepting the gift, then he or she should follow their instincts and refuse the gift. If it does not feel appropriate to accept the gift, then it probably isn't. It is difficult to imagine a circumstance in which a nurse might accept a gift of great value as the more expensive the gift, the greater the potential for misunderstanding.

WILLS

Due to the nature and length of the relationship between community nurses and their patients, the nurse may be asked to witness a will. It is perfectly acceptable, under law, for nurses to witness the will of one of their patients, unless they stand to benefit under the will. However, the employing health authority or Trust may have policies that prevent staff from acting as witnesses to wills. Although this may seem harsh, it often makes sense for nurses not to witness the wills of their patients.

There are strict rules governing the making of wills; if these rules are not followed the will may be invalid or open to challenge in court. Unless they know the rules nurses may inadvertently invalidate a will. Also, it is possible that if a will is challenged, the nurse, acting as witness, may be called to give evidence in court. This will result in the nurse being away from work, perhaps for a significant amount of time in complicated cases.

Check the employer's policies on witnessing of wills; some will have solicitors who will advise employees. Do not think that by witnessing a will you are necessarily doing a service for your patient.

Conclusion

The purpose of ethics and law in relation to health care is to protect patients' rights as well as those of nurses. The nurse who understands and follows the ethical and legal considerations presented above, will be providing a service to the patient that is founded upon a solid professional framework, a framework that will provide the patient with the standard of care they deserve, and nurses with the professional freedom that they need to develop and enhance their practice.

References

Beauchamp, T. and Childress, J. (1994) *Principles of biomedical ethics* (fourth edition). New York: Oxford University Press.

Curzon, L. (1996) *Dictionary of law*. London: Pitman Publishing.

Department of Health (DOH). (1995) *The patient's charter*. London: DOH.

Kant, I. (1973) *Immanuel Kant's critique of pure reason*. (Translated by Norman Smith Hampshire.) London: Macmillan.

Kennedy, I. and Grubb, A. (1994) *Medical law – text with materials*. London: Butterworths.

Kennedy, I. and Grubb, A. (1998) *Principles of medical law*. Oxford: Oxford University Press.

Montgomery, J. (1997) *Health care law*. Oxford: Oxford University Press.

United Kingdom Central Council (UKCC). (1992a) *Code of professional conduct*. London: UKCC.

United Kingdom Central Council (UKCC). (1992b) *Scope of professional practice*. London: UKCC.

United Kingdom Central Council (UKCC). (1966) *Guidelines for professional practice*. London: UKCC.

10 Evidence-based practice, clinical governance and community nurses

Val Woodward

Introduction

This chapter explores the concept of evidence-based practice and how this affects the community nurse practising in an environment increasingly influenced by governmental policies seeking efficiency and effectiveness, and the evidence-based movement with increasingly highlighted as the way forward for all healthcare professions. The term 'community nurses' in this chapter covers all disciplines of qualified nurses and health visitors who work in a community setting.

As far back as 1972 the Briggs report (DHSS, 1972) advised that nursing should become a research-based profession. However, it has taken over 20 years for these principles of research-mindedness to be adopted throughout nursing policy and practice. The 1990s have seen many changes to the National Health Service (NHS) research strategy as a whole. The Department of Health (DOH) strategy, *Research for Health* (DOH, 1991) required that research and development should become an integral part of health care, with all practitioners using research to inform decision-making. *The Report of the Taskforce on the Strategy for Research in Nursing, Midwifery and Health Visiting* (DOH, 1993), recommended the facilitation of increased amounts of higher quality research, and enhancement of nurses' research skills and experience in order to increase involvement in research.

Since the Culyer report (DOH, 1994), reorganization of the way research and development activity is funded and administered within the NHS has occurred. In addition, clinical governance has become a central part of the present government's policy, and embraces clinical effectiveness and efficiency, quality and accountability, with the setting up of systems for monitoring and evaluating these aspects of care (NHS Executive, 1999). These policies affect primary care groups (PCGs) and primary care trusts (PCTs) as well as other NHS Trusts, which are charged with putting into place systems for implementing and monitoring clinical governance. All practitioners are now expected to use evidence to justify decisions as part of the clinical governance framework, and to use evidence-based frameworks, guidelines and protocols for many aspects of care.

What is evidence-based practice?

The evidence-based practice movement has arisen from the move in medicine towards delivery of care based on evidence. Foundations for this were laid by Archie Cochrane, a medical practitioner who recognized a gap in medical evidence, namely a lack of critical summaries of randomized controlled trials (Cochrane, 1972). A shift away from basing decisions on opinion, past practice and precedent has been made in favour of using science, research and evidence to guide decision-making. Evidence-based medicine involves the application of clinical trial evidence to everyday practice (Baker *et al.*, 1997) and has been defined as:

> The conscientious, explicit and judicious use of current best evidence in making decisions about the care of individual patients. The practice of evidence-based medicine means integrating individual clinical expertise with the best available external evidence from systematic research.
> (Sackett *et al.*, 1996: 71)

The term 'evidence-based practice' has been defined as:

> An approach to decision making in which the clinician uses the best evidence available, in consultation with the patient, to decide upon the option which suits that patient best.
> (Muir Gray, 1997: 9)

There is now a firm commitment to an evidence-based NHS (DOH, 1996a, 1997), with the formation of national frameworks to support this such as a National Register of Research, the Cochrane Centre and database, and the NHS Centre for Reviews and Dissemination (Mulhall and Le May, 1999).

When transferring the concept of evidence-based practice to other disciplines, it has been recognized that evidence from randomized trials is not going to be available as a basis for all clinical decisions. The important point is to be able to identify the nature of the evidence-base that informs decisions (DOH, 1996b).

Applying the concept of evidence-based practice to nursing

A hierarchy of evidence has arisen within evidence-based medicine, with randomized controlled trials being seen as the 'gold standard' for all evidence.

Five categories of evidence have been identified and placed in descending order of value (Muir Gray, 1997):

- Systematic reviews and meta-analyses of multiple randomised controlled trials.
- Single randomized controlled trial.
- Non-randomized controlled trials, cohort or case-control studies.
- Non-experimental studies from more than one centre or research group.
- Opinion of respected authorities, based on clinical evidence, descriptive studies, or reports of expert committees.

The development of a hierarchy of evidence in medicine has added a 'currency' value to types of knowledge, placing empirical knowledge in the form of experimentation at the top of the tree. There is much debate, as to the worth of this currency in nursing: the complexities of nursing practice have led to dissatisfaction with the medical approach to evidence (Kendall, 1997; Wilson-Barnett, 1997; Clarke, 1999; Le May, 1999).

This hierarchical approach has advantages when considering, for example, new drug therapies, but its application to nursing, midwifery and health visiting can be seen to have limitations. The consideration of a broader base of knowledge is more applicable; nursing is a human-orientated practice with many dimensions. For example, a nurse who is making a decision as to which wound dressing is best for a particular client needs to consider a variety of factors such as:

- Type and condition of wound and surrounding skin.
- Co-existing medical conditions.
- Client mobility.
- Social and psychological factors.
- Response to previous treatments.
- Research evidence demonstrating efficacy of proposed dressing(s).
- Which dressings are available on prescription.
- Patient preferences.

It is not simply a matter of which product performed best in randomized controlled trials; this information should be considered as part of the over-all decision, but other factors play a considerable part in the final choice. However, community nurses need to be aware of the need for accurate documentation, and record all the factors considered in order to justify their decisions.

It can be seen from the above example that when considering types of evidence relevant to nursing decisions, knowledge from sources other than primary research is often utilized. There are several differing types of knowledge available on which to base these decisions (Figure 10.1).

The recognition by government that evidence from randomized controlled trials is not going to be sufficient as a basis for all clinical decisions for non-medical professions (DOH, 1996b) shows that the concept of evidence-based practice is constantly being developed and refined away from the narrow model used in medicine. James and Smith (1999) suggest

Theoretical knowledge is frequently linked to knowledge which is not generated through research or practice, but through a process of logical thought. In some instances you may find theoretical knowledge linked with the testing or generating of theories through research

Empirical knowledge is generated through research

Practical knowledge emanates from practice: it may be generated through research or logical thought associated with practice. many, however, would say that this type of knowledge emerges from the practice of nursing, midwifery and health visiting

Experiential knowledge is accumulated through our day-to-day experiences associated with our professional and personal lives

Interpersonal knowledge is linked with experiential knowledge but is associated with knowledge gained through interacting with people. This type of knowledge is particularly important within nursing, midwifery and health visiting since our practice revolves around interactions with others (patients/clients, carers, peers, other professionals)

Rituals is often associated with the traditions of practice and may provide a protective backdrop for care. All too often, however, the effectiveness of our rituals is unquestioned and unevaluated

Intuitive knowledge is hard to define. Frequently we cannot give an explanation for it other than 'we just knew' – it appears to be the ability to come to a decision without logical thought.

Figure 10.1   Types of knowledge (Le May, 1999)

that nurses use an alternative meaning for the word 'scientific': that of 'assisted by expert knowledge', in order to '... ground our examination of what is scientific about nursing practice in a thorough investigation of the expert knowledge held by health care professionals in a variety of settings' (p. 199).

Sources of evidence

When considering sources of evidence, it is necessary to look at a variety of information that reflects the type of knowledge-base. There is an increasing amount of written information available to practitioners from libraries, and electronic sources such as the Internet and CD-ROMs are expanding rapidly.

Sources of written information include:

- Journals.
- Books.
- Reviews.
- Government publications.
- Electronic databases, such as Cumulative Index to Nursing and Allied Health Literature (CINAHL), MEDLINE, English National Board Health Care Database, Bath Information and Data Services (BIDS), Applied Social Science Index and Abstracts (ASSIA), PsycLIT, Excerpta Medica (EmBASE), Allied and Alternative Medicine (AMED), Cochrane Library and National Research Register (NRR).
- 'Grey' literature – unpublished work, such as theses, dissertations, unpublished research or audit results.
- Guidelines and protocols – national and/or local.

Such sources are increasing rapidly and this list is not exhaustive. Non-written sources of evidence include:

- Conferences and seminars.
- Expert opinion, for example, national committees, working parties and task forces.
- Networks, support groups, professional organizations.
- Local knowledge and experience.

With such a vast amount of information available, it is often argued that it is impossible to keep up to date with and access new information and research. For community nurses this can be particularly relevant; they may work far away from large centres of information, unlike nurses working in a large hospital where there is often access to an NHS library, computers, the Internet and so on. These problems can be eased if community nurses are attached to a health centre or GP practice where computing facilities are available. One survey found that 20% of GPs had access to bibliographic databases in their surgeries, and 17% had access to the Internet (McColl *et al.*, 1998). These numbers are rapidly increasing as GP practices are now linking to the National Electronic Library for Health, part of the information management and technology network, a nationwide system that is part of the clinical governance initiative. It is a requirement (NHS Executive, 1998) that all GP practices will eventually be linked to these networks. These systems have Internet access, from which electronic searches can be made. Practices may also be linked to databases such as MEDLINE, as any member of the British Medical Association (BMA) is entitled to free membership of this particular database (Baker *et al.*, 1997). Community nurses need to ascertain exactly what facilities are available in their areas and negotiate access with appropriate parties.

It is increasingly important for community nurses to learn how to perform an electronic search and use a database; as search skills increase it becomes an easy way of accessing research abstracts and, in some cases, complete papers. Publications now give guidance to help novice searchers develop their skills in detail (see, for example, Greenhalgh, 1997). However, it is recognized that electronic searching does not provide a completely accurate service; hand searching can produce articles and papers not found by electronic means. For example, MEDLINE and EmBASE cover only about 6000 of the 20 000 relevant journals published world-wide (Muir Gray, 1997). When information is sought this should be borne in mind. Rights of access to local NHS or university libraries can be explored; many university or NHS libraries will allow community nurses to use their facilities for reference purposes, even if full lending rights are denied.

Making sense of the literature

The vast amount of health-related research now undertaken has led to the formation of national centres to undertake critical appraisal and systematic reviews, in order to provide community nurses with up-to-date knowledge of best available evidence about aspects of health care.

A systematic review is an overview of primary research studies on a set topic that contains an explicit statement of objectives, materials and methods, and has been conducted using explicit and reproducible methodology (Cochrane Collaboration, 1997). It has the advantage of limiting bias, providing accurate, reliable results and assimilating large amounts of information in a single paper. Systematic reviews can be either qualitative, providing a narrative review, or quantitative, providing a statistical analysis of all the eligible data. The latter type, known as a meta-analysis, is frequently used to review experimental research such as randomized controlled trials, and provides a statistical synthesis of the numerical results of several trials that all examined the same question (Greenhalgh, 1997). This increases the precision of the overall result.

The importance given to such reviews seems to have carried through an emphasis on medical research rather than nursing research: the meta-analysis, in particular, concentrates on experimental research methodology, which is found frequently in medicine but far less frequently in nursing research. Systematic reviews of qualitative research are rare, and this presents a dilemma: nursing research uses a wide range of designs which include many qualitative methods, and if the current emphasis on the importance of systematic reviews is to continue, more reviews of those areas that are often investigated qualitatively need to be undertaken and added to the national databases. If this is not done, a selection bias will occur in the type of research available for use in practice, and a great deal of important information will be lost. This will, in turn, have implications for the type of research that is funded and undertaken by nurses.

The national databases include the NHS Centre for Reviews and Dissemination (NHS CRD) and the Cochrane Centre, which were established in the 1990s to provide systematic reviews using a number of strategies. The Cochrane Centre led to the formation of an international movement, the Cochrane Collaboration, that reviews and disseminates international research and promotes fields of healthcare, of which primary health care is one. The NHS CRD maintains two databases: the Database of Abstracts of Reviews of Effectiveness (DARE), and the NHS Economic Evaluation Database, as well as undertaking or commissioning systematic reviews, and disseminating the results of reviews to the NHS. The Centre for Evidence-Based Nursing has been established under the NHS R&D programme, and is based at the University of York to provide systematic reviews of nursing and identify areas where research is needed. The National Institute for Clinical Excellence (NICE) has been established to promote clinical and cost-effectiveness, and will produce and disseminate high-quality, evidence-based guidance to support practitioners, including guidelines for the management of diseases and the use of significant new and existing interventions (NHS Executive, 1999).

The increasing development of systematic reviews of research on a national and international scale will influence the way community nurses practice. It is no longer acceptable to rely on ritual and tradition; they are expected to provide appropriate evidence to justify decisions. This includes keeping up to date with high-quality research findings, and the provision of good systematic reviews will aid this process by providing empirical evidence to complement the knowledge base. Community nurses need to ensure that they have access to appropriate evidence, understand it, are able to appraise it critically, and then apply it to their practice as appropriate.

Evidence-based practice, PCGs/PCTs and clinical governance

Recent changes in primary care, with the setting up of PCGs, are discussed in detail in Chapter 1. PCGs have replaced the previous fundholding/non-fundholding systems in general practice, and the purchaser—provider philosophy between Trusts. They provide a lead role in the planning, provision and development of local health services, acting as subcommittees of the local health authority with PCGs at Level 2 holding about 70% of the total general medical services budget. The main functions of PCGs are to improve the health and reduce health inequalities of the local community, develop primary care and community services, commission a range of hospital and community services which meet patients needs and introduce the clinical governance agenda to practices. They cover all GPs and patients within their geographical boundary. There are four levels of responsibility, and some PCGs have already progressed to PCT status, working at Level 4 as independent bodies taking responsibility for all services including full budgetary control.

Each PCG/PCT is required to appoint a Board member (usually a doctor but with potential for collaboration or joint sharing with a nurse) as the lead clinician to take responsibility for the concept of clinical governance. The Labour government has placed great emphasis on improving the quality of patient care in the NHS as set out in *The New NHS – Modern and Dependable*

(DOH, 1997) and in *A First Class Service: Quality in the new NHS* (DOH, 1998a). The term 'clinical governance' is defined as 'A framework through which NHS organizations are accountable for continuously improving the quality of their services and safeguarding high standards of care by creating an environment in which excellence in clinical care will flourish' (NHS Executive, 1999). It can be seen that research and evidence-based practice will be a major component of this framework: quality patient care can be promoted by the incorporation of practice based on best evidence of effectiveness. If a particular aspect of care is not proven to be effective, it should not be provided, but replaced with one that has been shown by research to be effective.

The main components of clinical governance are:

- Clear lines of responsibility and accountability for the overall quality of care.
- A comprehensive programme of quality improvement activities.
- Clear policies aimed at managing risks.
- Effective procedures to identify and remedy poor performance.

In order to achieve this, the clinical governance lead clinician has to ensure that correct processes are put and kept in place for monitoring and improving the quality of health care that the PCG/PCT provides and ensuring personal and organizational regulation of professionals. All general practices have had to nominate a clinical governance lead within the practice who liaises with the PCG/PCT lead. PCG/PCTs must demonstrate features such as:

- An open and participative culture in which education, research and the sharing of good practice are valued and expected.
- A commitment to quality supported by clearly identified local resources.
- A tradition of active working with patients, users, carers and the public.
- An ethos of multidisciplinary team working at all levels.
- Regular Board-level discussion of all major quality issues.
- Good use of information to plan and assess progress (NHS Executive, 1999).

The use of terms such as 'research', 'good practice', 'quality' and 'good use of information' all highlight the move towards an evidence-based climate. Some see the advent of clinical governance as a response to recent disasters in medical care, for example, relating to cervical screening, breast screening, the Bristol children's cardiac surgery case, and aspects of psychiatric care provision (Lugon and Secker-Walker, 1999). Critics of the clinical governance framework worry that an atmosphere of regulation and tighter control may be introduced at the expense of trust and culture (Davies and Mannion, 1999). Others suggest that it is yet another tactic to distract clinicians from issues such as increasingly centralized control and tight budgetary limitations, commenting on the lack of resources available to deliver high-quality care and support improvements (Frazer, 1998; Richards, 1998). However, it has been given a cautious welcome by many practitioners, with some noting that it largely clarifies and structures activities that have always been regarded as the foundations of good professional practice (Davies and Mannion, 1999). Clinical governance should act as a constant reminder of what is best practice, and focus the attention of community nurses on their own individual practice as well as the practices of their organizations as a whole.

Main components of clinical governance

How then does clinical governance relate to community nurses and primary health care generally? The government has outlined the main components of clinical governance (NHS Executive, 1999: 23–5). These are as follows.

CLEAR LINES OF RESPONSIBILITY AND ACCOUNTABILITY FOR THE OVERALL QUALITY OF CLINICAL CARE

A formal clinical governance committee is responsible within NHS Trusts, PCGs and PCTs for overseeing the process. It will provide regular reports to the governing Board on the quality of clinical care given, and produce an annual report of the programme as a whole. These regular reports are to be given the same importance as monthly financial reports. A designated senior clinician is responsible for co-ordinating this process and monitoring effectiveness; regular reporting mechanisms are being put in place. In NHS Trusts and PCTs, the chief executives carry ultimate responsibility for assuring quality of services provided. This is a new development: in the past, no one single person has been ultimately responsible for the quality of services provided by the organization.

A COMPREHENSIVE PROGRAMME OF QUALITY IMPROVEMENT ACTIVITIES

This includes routinely applying evidence-based practice to everyday care. Local PCGs and Trusts will identify and provide structures to implement and monitor national service frameworks and long-term service agreements, and community nurses will be expected to base their practice on recognized guidelines, systematic reviews, and information from organizations such as NICE.

Facilities are becoming available for all practitioners to access electronic databases, driven by the national information management (IM) and information technology (IT) strategy (NHS Executive, 1998), and community nurses will be expected to utilize these to gain the knowledge and evidence needed to improve the quality of their work. IT facilities, such as the Internet, telemedicine, satellite facilities, electronic mail and voice mail, will be incorporated as part of the wider communication network, with all practices using computer systems for data recording. Increasingly, community nurses will be expected to use these technologies: how well prepared are they for these changes? Training needs in these areas of practice, will need to be identified and acted upon.

Community nurses will, increasingly, be expected to work as part of a multidisciplinary and also a multi-agency team as it is recognized that many patients' needs derive from chronic diseases that require care from a range of health professionals working in different organizations within a locality. Examples include the care of patients with diseases such asthma, diabetes and epilepsy. PCGs and Trusts will be expected to link services to identified health needs in their local health improvement programme (HImP). These clinical teams will be expected to commission, analyse and assess the quality of services and seek ways to improve them in collaboration with other professionals such as public health teams, epidemiologists, statisticians and so on. Traditional tools, such as audit and research, will be used as evidence, and will gather information on effectiveness and outcomes.

The term 'seamless approach' has been adopted for high-quality care delivered by multisectoral, multiprofessional groups. Integrated care pathways are gaining popularity, and are often designed for a particular disease rather than a population. Nurses should be involved in designing these pathways, and they need to identify the extent of their own skills-base in this field. The use of evidence to formulate these pathways will be an important aspect of maintaining clinical governance across the primary/secondary interface, and the effectiveness of these can be monitored to reveal any gaps in care. It is likely that these results will be fed back to teams and individual practitioners who will then need to justify any deviation from the recommended pathway.

Programmes aimed at meeting the continuing professional development needs of individuals to improve quality are being put in place by PCGs and the Trusts in which community nurses work. Eventually, educational needs will be assessed via the PCGs if they reach Trust status to become PCTs. PCTs will notify the local education-purchasing consortium of specific needs for educational provision; these consortia provide the funding for educational development. PCTs will then be responsible for controlling and allocating allotted funding and undertaking workforce planning for this process, and may in the future employ most community practitioners in their area.

The PCTs will need to be seen to be fair in this process, and procedures for annual appraisal of staff, individual professional development plans, and practice development plans are already being implemented. These will enable individual practitioners and teams to identify developmental and educational needs that are directly related to the improvement of patient care and patient services. Certain groups of community nurses may benefit from this process: practice nurses, in particular, are at present at the dictates of their GP employers as to how much and what type of educational and developmental activities they undertake. However, it remains to be seen how far budgetary restrictions will affect this process: if there are large numbers of community nurses within a PCT, competition for resources may be intense.

It will be interesting to monitor how much of the educational budget is spent on the enhancement of research appreciation and appraisal skills, as opposed to clinical courses. PCTs and education purchasing consortia will be expected to work closely with education providers, such as universities, to ensure that courses are available that are linked to local health needs as identified in the HImPs, or to meet identified staff developmental needs. This may require increasing flexibility on behalf of the education providers to respond to specific areas of demand for education not traditionally offered, but may be at the expense of providing the skills and education needed to ensure that practice is firmly underpinned by research and evidence.

Documentation of care will increasingly play a major role as community nurses are expected to justify clinical decisions and provide evidence to support care and treatment proposed or given. This will be achieved via effective monitoring of clinical care using high-quality systems for clinical record keeping and the collection of relevant information. The IM and IT strategy is looking towards complete electronic patient health records in the next three to five years (NHS Executive, 1998). Appropriate safeguards to protect access to and storage of confidential patient information are to be monitored, and community nurses will have to ensure that they are aware of local policy with regard to access, storage and transport of patient records. Quality assurance processes will be in place and integrated within the quality programme of organizations as a whole: community nurses may be involved in gathering information and evidence, setting standards and monitoring outcomes in their particular fields to feed into organizational processes. Trusts are now being directed to undertake an annual record/documentation audit.

Quality improvement activities should also encourage participation in well-designed, relevant research and development (R&D) activity that contributes to the development of an evaluation culture. Trusts and PCGs will be expected to encourage these projects, and community practitioners with an interest in this area should be supported by their organizations. Up to now, there has been very little R&D money in the primary care system. Most R&D funding was allocated to the acute sectors, with only very small amounts going to primary care. Very little has been allocated to nurses. This raises issues of inequality and problems with improvements in care. If research funding is limited, opportunities for developing services and care will be constrained.

However, this is being recognized, and the latest review of R&D funding (DOH, 2000) aims to minimize bureaucracy for those pursuing R&D in primary care and develop and support this research. The DOH is working with the Federation of Primary Care Research Networks to agree core network and practice activities, and associated costs that are eligible for R&D funding under the new 'Priorities and Needs' fund. These primary care research networks exist to provide an opportunity for practitioners working in primary care to meet, exchange views, hear presentations of existing research projects, undertake research and learn more about research methods. They are an ideal way for community nurses to become more aware of research activity in their areas, to network with other community practitioners with an interest in R&D, and keep up to date with developments in primary care research. The DOH is also planning to develop criteria, to identify primary care sites that collaborate with research or undertake research, in order for appropriate funding to be available to meet costs incurred in supporting and managing R&D. This funding will be available from the 'Support for Science' arm of funding (DOH, 2000).

CLEAR POLICIES AIMED AT MANAGING RISKS

Organizations should promote self-assessment to identify and manage risk. The principal aim of risk management is to reduce the chance of patients being harmed, but risk management will also reduce the risk of complaints or litigation against community nurses or their organizations (Roland and Baker, 1999). It will encompass a range of activities that aim to develop good practice and prevent harmful or adverse events happening.

Both personal clinical responsibilities, and the need for effective systematic reduction of risk, are incorporated. Organizational risk management has been introduced to ensure that organizations are well managed; the task of delivering high-quality care is easier if organizations have in place sound financial systems and complementary arrangements for assessing and managing organizational risks, for example, those that affect the health and safety of patients and staff, and dealing with complaints. The personal responsibilities of community include nurses anticipating and preventing potential problems, learning from critical incidents and patient complaints and using systems to reflect upon and develop their practice.

Ways in which community nurses could achieve this include being aware of the rationale of risk management and their organizations' policies (for example, complaints procedures and reporting systems); using evidence to inform practice (for example from organizations such as NICE and the Cochrane Library, or from local/national clinical guidelines, national service frameworks and so on); auditing their own practice and adjusting practice as identified by the audit cycle to demonstrate improvement; and using clinical supervision to reflect on individual strengths and examine personal development needs. These personal activities should link in with the wider organizational activities to provide a co-ordinated approach to risk management.

Risk management has not been traditionally well structured in the community and this is now being addressed. The Medical Defence Union (MDU) showed that the most common reasons for complaints in primary care were, in order: failure/delay in diagnosis; inadequate treatment/management; rude attitudes; failure/delay to visit; prescription problems; administration problems; and inadequate examination: the MDU concluded that the root cause for most complaints was a failure to communicate properly (Roland and Baker, 1999).

Risk management will be incorporated into everyday practice, and organizations should assess the systems in place to prevent errors such as those outlined above. The right systems need to be set up to reduce these risks and their effectiveness needs to be monitored.

PROCEDURES FOR ALL PROFESSIONAL GROUPS TO IDENTIFY AND REMEDY POOR PERFORMANCE

Such procedures include the reporting of critical incidents to ensure that adverse events are identified, with open investigations that provide opportunity for learning from mistakes and applying the lessons learned to practice. Formal complaints procedures need to be in place that are accessible to clients and their families and fair to staff. Lessons learned from the process should be used to avoid a recurrence of similar problems.

Procedures to monitor professional performance, such as annual appraisal, include all community practitioners, including GPs. These will ensure that potential problems are noted at an early stage before patients are harmed and are aimed at helping to improve practice. Areas of development identified at appraisal will be incorporated into personal development plans for the subsequent year. If there are any gaps in knowledge about evidence and best practice, they need to be identified at an early opportunity so that the personal development plan reflects this. All staff need to understand these procedures: they are accountable for their practice and need to demonstrate that their practice is based on best available evidence as part of the monitoring process. If this is not the case they are expected to identify the gaps in their knowledge and take steps to remedy them.

It is now recognized that all staff have areas of practice that they need to develop, and lifelong learning is encouraged. Clinical governance can thus be seen to be trying to move away from a climate of fear, by detecting problems at an early stage and aiming at staff development, rather than resorting to disciplinary measures. This should therefore encourage an open, facilitative approach that ensures that any problems are detected early and acted upon rather than being left to fester. These changes will affect community staff: for example, practice nurses are traditionally employed by GPs and have been used to performance issues being dealt with 'in-house'. Many have not had formal appraisals in the past. These changes will also have a significant effect upon GPs, as independent contractors, who are used to managing continuing professional development and clinical performance themselves. Peer review and clinical supervision are now mandatory for all doctors and nurses, and continuing professional development in general practice has been reviewed with major changes recommended to the way in which it is undertaken (DOH, 1998b). In future, it is likely that this will be managed in conjunction with PCGs/PCTs and monitored centrally. Some GPs view this as a threat to their independent status, but others believe that this centralization will achieve equality and standardization for all staff. A review of GPs involved in total purchasing revealed negative attitudes and concerns about clinical governance, but also showed a lack of understanding about its nature and implications (Malbon et al., 1998).

Staff with concerns about the professional performance and conduct of colleagues should be supported and encouraged to report such concerns and procedures for reporting are to be laid down. There is a clear message here that so-called 'whistle-blowers' should be able to report concerns without fear of retribution or worries about their own employment status. The Bristol Children's Hospital heart tragedy provides an example of the effects that reporting of concerns has had on individuals. The anaesthetist who reported his concerns over the outcomes of surgery had to leave the UK and seek work abroad as a result of making official his worries (Hammond and Mosley, 1999). This aspect of clinical governance aims to prevent victimization, and encourage openness about areas of concern, so that problems of this magnitude are never allowed to develop again.

The concept of evidence-based practice is an integral part of the clinical governance programme and threads through all aspects of the framework. Community nurses need to ensure that their clinical decisions are based on evidence that can be justified and demonstrated, and they will be held accountable for their decisions. Nurses are used to the notion of individual accountability with the development of the United Kingdom Central Council's (UKCC) *Code of Professional Conduct* (UKCC, 1984, 1992a) and the *Scope of Professional Practice* (UKCC, 1992b). Clinical governance takes the concept of accountability further to consider the wider organizational aspects, and sets out specific requirements that both organizations and individual practitioners need to address.

The focus of clinical governance is teamwork, partnership and communication. It will take time for a culture of quality improvement and evidence-based practice to become established. This is recognized by the government, which recommends key changes that will demonstrate in the short and medium term that clinical governance is being implemented successfully. Practitioners will need to be convinced that a balance is being achieved between checking and trusting. Measurement, monitoring and control are costly strategies; it remains to be seen how effective a strategy clinical governance will become.

Making evidence-based practice a reality

Community nurses need to be able to incorporate evidence into practice in order to provide a safe, effective service to clients and to meet the requirements of the clinical governance initiative. Sources of evidence have been explored previously: a topic has been identified, the evidence is there, the searches have been undertaken and the relevant evidence extracted. The next question is what to do with it.

First, the strengths and weaknesses of this evidence need to be appraised; the actual quality of evidence that is available is still not uniformly high, and practice should not be based on poor quality evidence. Second, a sophisticated approach to incorporating evidence and implementing evidence-based practice is needed, including an understanding of the context in which care is provided, and the obstacles which prevent individuals, teams and organizations from using evidence (Closs and Cheater, 1999).

APPRAISING THE EVIDENCE

Community nurses must develop the ability to appraise the research they read critically, in order to make informed decisions about the care that they give. Not all published research is rigorously planned, implemented and analysed, and they need to be able to sort out good quality, appropriate research from poor quality, or badly interpreted studies. It is not justifiable to change practice on the basis of poor quality or unreliable studies.

In order to appraise research critically, community nurses need to have an understanding of basic research methodology. This can be obtained by reading basic nursing research textbooks (see, for example, Cormack, 1996; Holloway and Wheeler, 1996; Bowling, 1997), attending workshops and study days, for example those organized locally by research and development support units and trusts, and/or attendance on modules offered by higher education institutes, for example a research methods course accredited at diploma level (Level 2) or higher as appropriate for individual needs. Such modules are proving increasingly popular as both practitioners and managers recognize the importance of nurses developing their research skills and knowledge, and can usually be taken as 'stand-alone' modules as well as part of academic courses. At the University of Plymouth, for example, the Institute of Health Studies offers a basic research methods module at Level 2: this is now the most-purchased module in the Institute, demonstrating the increasing awareness of practitioners and managers of the importance of this knowledge.

Appraisal checklists can be found in nursing and research textbooks (e.g. Sackett et al., 1991; Cormack, 1996; Crombie, 1996; Greenhalgh, 1997) and programmes have been devised to provide training in critical appraisal skills, such as the Critical Appraisal Skills Programme (CASP), an Oxford-based workshop approach that introduces participants to the identification and appraisal of research into the effectiveness of health care. The CASP programme provides a web site for further information at http://www.ihs.ox.ac.uk/casp/ Critical appraisal modules can also be accessed from universities, either as discrete modules, or incorporated into research methods courses as described above.

Appraisal checklists will look at areas such as the processes involved, methods used, rigour of the research (to include reliability and validity in quantitative papers, and trustworthiness in qualitative papers), the analysis of results and conclusions drawn. The emphasis on what to look for will vary according to the type of research; publications provide appropriate guidance for appraising a variety of methodologies to include surveys, randomized controlled trials, cohort studies, case-control studies, reviews, guidelines, economic analyses and qualitative studies (see, for example, Crombie, 1996; Greenhalgh, 1997; Muir Gray, 1997). When appraising a number of papers about the same topic, it can be useful to prepare a matrix using several appraisal criteria in order to compare the results if a good quality systematic review of the literature has not already been undertaken (see Roe, 1993: 38–9). This will enable comparisons to be made, not only of the content and findings but also of the rigour with which methodological aspects were undertaken. This will then make the process of deciding whether or not the research merits a change in practice much easier and more structured, so that good quality research is recognized and implemented, without the danger of poor quality research being used to influence practice.

Community nurses should always establish whether a good quality systematic review or meta-analysis has been undertaken in the field; these provide concentrated sources of evidence that can save time and provide an appraisal of several papers on the same topic. National guidelines also need to be identified if they exist, as they can provide a template for planning changes to practice. For example, asthma management is clearly laid out in the British Thoracic Society (BTS) guidelines (British Thoracic Society, National Asthma Campaign, Royal College of Physicians of London, 1997). These guidelines were devised using evidence from a variety of sources, and put together by a panel of experts in the field. They have standardized the management of asthma, and provide a framework for the development of local policies and protocols to reflect local needs.

IDENTIFYING AND COPING WITH BARRIERS TO CHANGE

Implementing research and applying evidence to practice is not an easy task. You have identified an area in need of investigation, updated your skills, found and appraised the relevant evidence and identified a need for a change in practice. However, finding ways to incorporate the evidence seems difficult. This is not surprising: numerous barriers to using evidence have been identified by research (Veeramah, 1995; Hunt, 1996; Le May, 1999) and include the following:

- Resistance to change.
- Lack of resources.
- Lack of organizational support.
- Lack of time.
- Attitudes of colleagues – both nursing and other professionals.
- Conflicting evidence.
- Ambiguous findings.
- Lack of knowledge to appraise research or implement research findings.
- Inability to access research evidence.

There are ways to approach these problems. For example, it is often much easier to implement the evidence if the whole team is involved with the process. This could be achieved in several ways such as setting up a journal club, as part of clinical supervision, or through team meetings or a steering group. It can be made far less stressful and encourages teamwork to undertake this with colleagues, for example identifying issues needing attention, all looking for appropriate literature, studying the research together and meeting as a team to consider the findings and their relevance to their particular area. If all team members can see the need for change, and are involved in the process, it becomes needs-led and 'bottom-up' rather than being seen as imposed from management. The chances of succeeding are then much greater. Sound communication skills are required for this process. However, wider organizational issues need to be considered as part of this process, and inclusion of managers and relevant personnel such as other community practitioners, doctors, professions allied to medicine (and external agencies such as social services if appropriate) at this stage may avoid problems later in the process. Barriers to their particular project need to be identified by the team at the outset so that ways to overcome them can be addressed.

ORGANIZATIONAL CHANGE AND SUPPORT

In order to utilize evidence, changes to practice will need to be undertaken. The management of change within the organization needs to be considered, as well as the effects of change on individuals. Changes may be needed to the way in which services are arranged: equipment used may need reviewing or altering, staffing arrangements may need to change and there may be alterations in professional boundaries (Mulhall, 1999); for example, more equality between doctors and nurses, or more commonality between community nursing specialisms. Time and resources will need to be identified to support staff development, provide equipment and undertake an evaluation such as audit of outcomes.

The new responsibilities of organizations now mandatory within the clinical governance framework may, however, provide an ideal catalyst for changes that improve the utilization of evidence, and community nurses should seize the opportunity to look closely at their practice, their organizations and their responsibility to provide care based on best-available evidence. Lewin (1951) devised a force-field theory of change that looked at forces driving change and forces resisting change. He proposed a three-phase model for change: unfreezing (becoming aware of the need for change), working on the change (planning and introducing change, reducing resisting forces), and refreezing (incorporating the change into everyday activities, so that it becomes normal practice). Mulhall (1999) warns, however, that effective and sustainable change to nursing practice will only occur with:

- A framework that incorporates awareness of how the social structure of the NHS affects change.
- A clearer statement of the evidence that nursing needs for effective practice.
- A strategy and context that provides adequate resources to effect change.

Several large-scale projects have investigated the utilization of research evidence in practice. Examples include the Conduct and Utilization of Research in Nursing (CURN) project (Michigan Nurses Association, 1983), and the Getting Research into Purchasing and Practice (GriPP) project introduced by Anglia and Oxford Regional Health Authority in 1993 to focus on interventions for which there was good research evidence of effectiveness, but where a gap existed between this evidence and what was done in practice (Anglia and Oxford Regional Health Authority, 1994). The Framework for Appropriate Care Throughout Sheffield (FACTS) project commenced in 1994, concentrating on GP practices, aiming to change behaviour so that it became more evidence-based (Eve, 1995). Papers by Funk *et al.* (1989), and Closs and Cheater (1994) and French (1999) also look at dissemination and/or utilization of research.

However, willingness to change does not always guarantee success, for example, many health visiting students in the University of Plymouth each year develop a protocol for introducing the use of the Edinburgh Post-natal Depression Scale (EPDS) (Cox *et al.*, 1987) into practice. This scale has been shown to be highly effective in identifying postnatal depression (Briscoe, 1989; Clifford *et al.*, 1999), but is still not routinely used by all organizations or practitioners. I myself have worked with one trust to develop a strategy for nursing research and development which initially faltered due to lack of funding to provide a research and development nurse to support practitioners. The will was there but the finance was not. Organizational change is perhaps the hardest thing to achieve, and it may be better to first look closely at small projects that are achievable rather than to try to scale Everest straight away. Figure 10.2 provides some clinical scenarios as examples for a range of community specialisms, and some of the questions that community nurses should be asking themselves when considering whether their care is based on evidence.

Action research can be used as a method of achieving change in practice: one of the aims of action research is to create change and improve practice. The approach is a problem solving one that involves collaboration between researcher and practitioner, with the identification and resolution of problems, changes in behaviour, and theory construction (Hart and Bond, 1995). The researcher acts as facilitator, and works with practitioners rather than doing research 'on' them and reflective practice is encouraged as a means to identify problems. Known local researchers could be approached if readers are interested in this method.

Increasingly, organizations are developing strategies to manage and organize research activity, and all such activity now has to be monitored and documented centrally to fulfil the requirements of the Culyer report (DOH, 1994). Many organizations are employing designated research and development nurses and practice development nurses. Community nurses need to ascertain what their particular organizational strategy is, and who they can contact for advice and support. Designated staff are there to provide support for practitioners, and changing practice to utilize evidence is an area that can be undertaken in conjunction with such advisors. Organizations that are too small to have designated departments, such as GP practices, will still have to incorporate the clinical governance framework. Local PCG/PCTs will provide guidance and support to practices and community nurses should ascertain who provides this support. Changes in GP practices need to be undertaken in conjunction with the rest of the practice and primary health care team: they may not only impinge on the GPs but also on receptionists, practice managers, and community practitioners working in or attached to the practice, such as health visitors, practice nurses, midwives and district nurses.

Ear syringing

When ears are to be syringed, what agent do I recommend for softening wax? How long do I recommend its use and how often? What is the evidence for this? What is the most effective agent? Is water as effective? What side effects are there from the softening process? What type of equipment am I using to syringe the ears; are there any risks? What are the contraindications? Does the protocol I am using reflect the evidence?

Post-natal depression

Are there measures that are currently in place in my organization to detect post-natal depression (PND)? What are they? Do I use them? Is there a protocol? Do these measures reflect the evidence? What is the most effective tool for detecting PND? Is the Edinburgh Post-natal Depression Scale recommended widely? Should it be used routinely for all post-natal mothers? If so, when and how often? Should it be used ante-natally to identify possible risk?

School entry health promotion interviews at 11 years

Do I undertake a health promotion interview for individual students at secondary school entry? If not, would it be beneficial? Would it encourage improved access to drop-in services? Does it result in more effective health promotion experiences for the young people themselves? Could it target specific issues relevant to this age group more effectively than formal sessions in larger groups? Is it a useful preventative/early detection of problems service? What research has been done in this area? How could I set up such a service?

Severe mental health disorders – home or hospital?

Where is the best place for someone with severe mental health disorders to be cared for – at home or in hospital? What differences in outcomes are identified by research? What level of care is needed to provide a service in the community? Have I got the resources I need to provide this service? How are relatives affected? What support do I need to provide for them? What do patients prefer? What do relatives prefer?

Figure 10.2 Clinical scenarios for community nurses – considering the evidence, challenging practice

---

Terminally ill children – home or hospital?

What are the benefits for children with terminal illness of care at home as opposed to in hospital? What research has been undertaken in this field? What resources do I need to be able to provide this care? What type of support will I need to give parents/siblings/other family members? What other disciplines in the wider community could provide support for the family?

Behavioural problems in clients with learning disabilities

What care intervention is given to my clients with behavioural difficulties? Is it family therapy; cognitive behavioural therapy, other one-to-one intervention, anger management or something else? What is my rationale for choosing this intervention? Which of these have been shown to be effective? Have any been shown to be ineffective? What is the outcome of current care provision in this area for my clients? How has this been evaluated?

Figure 10.2 (Cont.)   Clinical scenarios for community nurses – considering the evidence, challenging practice

Organizations can also get help and advice from the Foundation of Nursing Studies (FNS), a charity involved in initiatives to support implementation and dissemination of research. The organization will fund projects that disseminate or implement proven research findings, organize conferences in partnership with NHS organizations, support networks and forums, provide workshops, and act in a consultancy role giving advice to NHS organizations (Mulhall and Le May, 1999). A series of FNS workshops for nurses, held in Plymouth in 1999, resulted in several practitioners or teams of practitioners implementing changes in practice to incorporate best evidence for the benefit of clients.

IMPLEMENTATION AND EVALUATION

When barriers have been identified and addressed, and organizational issues looked at, the means of implementation and evaluation needs to be decided. The style of implementation will obviously vary according to the nature of the project, but all team members need to be kept informed of how changes are to be introduced, and over what timescale. There are no set procedures for this, but methods of evaluating the outcomes need to be decided before the changes are implemented, and the planned changes should be seen as achievable by the team. It is better to plan small-scale changes to start with, evaluate and then move on if they are successful. In this way, positive outcomes are demonstrated and enthusiasm is maintained for further change.

Conclusions

This chapter has sought to give an overview of the nature of evidence, the concept of evidence-based practice, the clinical governance initiative and the relevance of these to community practitioners. Evidence-based practice is necessary if we are to provide clinically effective and cost-effective care to a growing population that is, increasingly, being cared for in the community. The nature of evidence is varied and may be derived from a variety of sources of knowledge; rigid definitions of evidence-based practice using a hierarchical approach (as in the medical model of evidence-based medicine) are inappropriate for the complexity of nursing activity.

As the need for care based on evidence has grown, centrally devised frameworks, via clinical governance, have been devised to provide a means of achieving care that is up to date, appropriate, and clinically and cost-effective. These frameworks are now being implemented and community nurses need to reflect on their practice and be aware of their responsibilities. Sophisticated approaches to implementing evidence-based practice are needed to include developing appraisal skills, acquiring an understanding of change mechanisms and barriers to change, and an appreciation of individual, team and organizational factors. Incorporating evidence into practice will take time, energy and support: it is to be hoped that the new policy framework of clinical governance will provide an incentive and also a supportive climate in which community nurses can develop their practice for the benefit of clients.

References

Anglia and Oxford Regional Health Authority (1994) *Getting research into practice and purchasing (GriPP). Four counties approach.* Oxford: NHS Executive Anglia and Oxford.

Baker, M., Maskrey, N. and Kirk, S. (1997) *Clinical effectiveness and primary care.* Abingdon: Radford Medical Press.

Bowling, A. (1997) *Research methods in health: investigating health and health services.* Buckingham: Open University Press.

Briscoe, M. (1989) The detection of emotional disorders in the post-natal period by health visitors. *Health Visitor*, 62: 340–2.

British Thoracic Society, National Asthma Campaign, Royal College of Physicians of London (1997) The British guidelines on asthma management. *Thorax*, 52 (Supplement 1): S1–S21.

Clarke, J.B. (1999) Evidence-based practice: a retrograde step? The importance of pluralism in evidence generation for the practice of health care. *Journal of Clinical Nursing*, 8: 89–94.

Clifford, C., Day, A., Cox, J. and Werrett, J. (1999) A cross-cultural analysis of the use of the Edinburgh Post-Natal Depression Scale (EPDS) in health visiting practice. *Journal of Advanced Nursing*, 30: 655–4.

Closs, S.J. and Cheater F.M. (1994) Utilization of nursing research: culture, interest and support. *Journal of Advanced Nursing*, 19: 762–73.

Closs, S.J. and Cheater, F.M. (1999) Evidence for nursing practice: a clarification of the issues. *Journal of Advanced Nursing*, 30: 10–17.

Cochrane, A.L. (1972) *Effectiveness and efficiency: random reflections on health services*. The Rock Carling Fellowship. Cambridge: Cambridge University Press.

Cochrane Collaboration (1997) *Cochrane Collaboration handbook*. (Database on disk and CD-Rom, available from Cochrane library) Issue 1. Oxford: Update Software.

Cormack, D.F.S. (ed) (1996) *The research process in nursing* (third edition). Oxford: Blackwell Science.

Cox, J.L., Holden, J.H. and Sagovsky, R. (1987) Detection of postnatal depression: development of the 10 item Edinburgh Postnatal Depression Scale. *British Journal of Psychiatry*, 150: 782–6.

Crombie, I.K. (1996) *The pocket guide to critical appraisal*. London: BMJ Publishing Group.

Davies, H.T.O. and Mannion, R. (1999) *Clinical governance: striking a balance between checking and testing. The York series on the NHS White Paper – a research agenda*. Discussion paper 165. York: Centre for Health Economics, University of York.

Department of Health (DOH). (1991) *Research for health: a research and development strategy for the NHS*. London: HMSO.

Department of Health (DOH). (1993) *Report of the taskforce on the strategy for research in nursing, midwifery and health visiting*. (Chairman, Adrian Webb) London: DOH.

Department of Health (DOH). (1994) *Supporting research and development in the NHS*. (Chairman, Anthony Culyer). London: HMSO.

Department of Health (DOH). (1996a) *Research and development: towards an evidence-based health service*. London: DOH.

Department of Health (DOH). (1996b) *Promoting clinical effectiveness: a framework for action in and through the NHS*. Leeds: NHS Executive.

Department of Health (DOH). (1997) *The new NHS – modern and dependable*. London: The Stationery Office.

Department of Health (DOH). (1998a) *A first class service: quality in the new NHS*. London: The Stationery Office.

Department of Health (DOH). (1998b) *A review of continuing professional development in general practice*. London: DOH.

Department of Health (DOH). (2000) *Research and development for a first class service: R&D funding in the new NHS*. London: DOH.

Department of Health and Social Security (DHSS). (1972) *Report of the committee on nursing*. (Chairman, Asa Briggs). London: HMSO.

Eve, R. (1995) *Implementing clinical change: learning from the US experience. FACTS programme*. Sheffield: University of Sheffield, Sheffield Centre for Health and Related Research.

Frazer, M. (1998) The government's initiative may be stillborn. *British Medical Journal*, 317: 687.

French, B. (1999) The dissemination of research. In: Mulhall, A. and Le May, A. (eds) *Nursing research: dissemination and implementation*. Edinburgh: Churchill Livingstone; 81–108.

Funk, S.G., Tornquist, E.M. and Champagne, M.T. (1989) A model for improving dissemination of nursing research. *Western Journal of Nursing Research*, 11: 361–7.

Greenhalgh, T. (1997) *How to read a paper: the basics of evidence-based medicine*. London: BMJ Publishing Group.

Hammond, P. and Mosley, M. (1999) *Trust me (I'm a doctor)*. London: Metro Books.

Hart, E. and Bond, M. (1995) *Action research for health and social care*. Buckingham: Open University Press.

Holloway, I. and Wheeler, S. (1996) *Qualitative research for nurses*. Oxford: Blackwell Science.

Hunt, J.M. (1996) Barriers to research utilisation. *Journal of Advanced Nursing*, 23: 423–5.

James, T. and Smith, P. (1999) Implementing research: the practice. In: Mulhall, A. and Le May, A. (eds) *Nursing research: dissemination and implementation*. Edinburgh: Churchill Livingstone; 177–204.

Kendall, S. (1997) What do we mean by evidence? Implications for primary health care nursing. *Journal of Interprofessional Care*, 11: 23–34.

Le May, A. (1999) Knowledge for dissemination and implementation. In: Mulhall, A. and Le May, A. (eds) *Nursing research: dissemination and implementation*. Edinburgh: Churchill Livingstone; 47–61.

Lewin, K. (1951) *Field theory in the social sciences*. New York: Harper.

Lugon, M. and Secker-Walker, J. (eds) (1999) *Clinical governance: making it happen*. London: Royal Society of Medicine.

Malbon, G., Gillan, S. and Mays, N. (1998) Clinical governance: onus points. *Health Service Journal*, 108: 28–9.

McColl, A., Smith, H., White, P. and Field, J. (1998) General practitioners' perceptions of the route to evidence-based medicine: a questionnaire survey. *British Medical Journal*, 316: 361–5.

Michigan Nurses Association (1983) *Conduct and utilization of research in nursing (CURN) project: using research to improve nursing practice*. Michigan: Grune & Stratton.

Muir Gray, J.A. (1997) *Evidence-based healthcare: how to make healthy policy and management decisions*. Edinburgh: Churchill Livingstone.

Mulhall, A. (1999) Creating change in practice. In: Mulhall, A. and Le May, A. (eds) *Nursing research: dissemination and implementation*. Edinburgh: Churchill Livingstone; 151–75.

Mulhall, A. and Le May, A. (eds) (1999) *Nursing research: dissemination and implementation*. Edinburgh: Churchill Livingstone.

NHS Executive (1998) *Information for health: an information strategy for the modern NHS 1998–2005*. Wetherby: NHS Executive.

NHS Executive (1999) *Clinical governance: quality in the new NHS*. Leeds: DOH.

Richards, P. (1998) Professional self respect: rights and responsibilities in the new NHS. *British Medical Journal*, 317: 1146–8.

Roe, B. (1993) Undertaking a critical review of the literature. *Nurse Researcher*, 1: 31–42.

Roland, M. and Baker, R. (1999) *Clinical governance: a practical guide for primary care teams*. Manchester: University of Manchester.

Sackett, D.L., Haynes, R.B., Guyatt, G.H. and Tugwee, P. (1991) *Clinical epidemiology: a basic science for clinical medicine*. Boston: Little Brown.

Sackett, D.L., Rosenberg, W.M.C., Muir Gray, J.A. *et al.* (1996) Evidence-based medicine: what it is and what it isn't. *British Medical Journal*, 312: 71–2.

United Kingdom Central Council for Nursing, Midwifery and Health Visiting (UKCC). (1984) *Code of professional conduct*. London: UKCC.

United Kingdom Central Council for Nursing, Midwifery and Health Visiting (UKCC). (1992a) *Code of professional conduct*. London: UKCC.

United Kingdom Central Council for Nursing, Midwifery and Health Visiting (UKCC). (1992b) *Scope of professional practice*. London: UKCC.

Veeramah, V. (1995) A study to identify the attitudes and needs of qualified staff concerning the use of research findings in clinical practice within mental health settings. *Journal of Advanced Nursing*, 22: 855–61.

Wilson-Barnett, J. (1997) Evidence for nursing practice – an overview. NT Research symposium for evidence-based nursing, Manchester. *NT Research*, 2: 12–14.

11 The development of community nursing in the light of the NHS Plan

Val Hyde and Clare Cotter

Introduction

From the first ten chapters in this book, it can be seen that community nurses are now working within an exciting context where the potential for role development and expansion is unprecedented; this role growth has been brought about by three things. First, new nurse-led primary care initiatives such as walk-in centres, have given rise to the creation of new roles. Second, roles which, until recently have been accepted and perpetuated as 'traditional', particularly those of doctors, are increasingly being adopted and practised by nurses. Third, large numbers of people who in the past, would have been cared for in other settings, are now remaining in their own homes, necessitating the design and delivery of increasingly complex and varied, packages of care.

In light of the above, this chapter will discuss some of the key factors that may influence the extent to which community nurses respond to the challenges presented and will consider, in the light of *The NHS Plan* (DOH, 2000a), issues that are of relevance to the development of community nursing, and the delivery of primary health care.

BOUNDARIES – MARKERS OF PROFESSIONAL TERRITORY?

Although it is encouraging that the full scope of community nurses' professional practice is at last being recognized and utilized, some personal reflection on the motivating impetus, is recommended. Could it be possible that, for some, extended boundaries signify more about the marking of further territory claimed for the profession than about the provision of a comprehensive, patient-centred service? Although pride in one's profession might cultivate a commitment to build a reputation of excellence and, therefore, effect an improvement in the quality of services, the latter is a secondary spin-off and clients are used as a means to promote the profession. If nurses concern themselves more with the profession's well-being and status than with the well-being of the clients/patients for whom the profession exists then their primary activity is the building of empires and the claim to professionalism is thereby undermined.

A pre-occupation with the promotion and protection of professional identity and status often leads to other behaviours that are neither becoming to professionals, nor advantageous to clients. For example, colleagues in other professional groups are perceived as competitors and opportunities are taken to criticize or devalue them. When addressing a conference of nurse leaders recently, Gough (cited in Donnelly, 2000a: 11) commented on the 'triumphalism about what is going on in the medical professions' that she had encountered in the preceding weeks, in her talks with nurses; she judged their attitude to be a 'very unhelpful way forward'.

BOUNDARIES – INTERPROFESSIONAL BARRIERS?

Nevertheless, various writers have noted the existence of such attitudes (Cumberlege, 1990; Dalley, 1993; Howkins, 1995) not only among nurses towards non-nurse colleagues but among social workers, health visitors, doctors and managers towards others with a different professional identity to their own. Indeed, despite the development of initiatives that have been established to dissolve barriers and promote joint learning and working between professions and individuals (for example, the Centre for the Advancement of Inter-professional Education) discussions about such barriers and their consequences, are still appearing in the literature with monotonous regularity and predictability:

- McDonald *et al.* (1997) draw attention to 'poor communication and animosity between different providers' which is seen as a 'stumbling block to the development of a workable and integrated service for the community' (p. 263).
- Castledine (1999) writes of roles and boundaries that need to be 'torn down' (p. 62) in order for multiprofessional dialogue to take place.
- Dixon (1998), comments on the 'exclusivity behaviours and power issues' (p. 282) that prevent effective shared learning (reporting on the CPHVA 'Partnerships in Practice Education' conference).
- Quinn (cited by Eaton, 1999: 8) expresses concern at the professional tribalism and vying for budgets, caused by the uncertainty of where nursing stops and social services start.
- Parkin (1999) refers to the 'negative stereotyping' of social workers by some GPs, district nurses and health visitors, 'based on a desire to protect professional boundaries' (p.23).
- Lockhart-Wood (2000: 280), in her study on collaboration between nurses and doctors in clinical practice, highlights as a major theme, the power imbalance that exists between the two, and the resultant dissatisfaction and frustration experienced by nurses.

These are just a few of a seemingly endless list; the reasons quoted for the existence of the barriers include political ideologies, socialization, etc. Castledine (2000) suggests a further reason: that against a backdrop of minimal control on how health services have evolved, 'the health professions themselves have tried to protect their own boundaries by becoming exclusive and resistant to external influences' (p. 382).

Whatever the reasons, those professionals who continue to perpetuate old prejudices and barriers do so at significant cost to the client. Unless they are enabled to change their perspectives and values, they will pose a threat to the success of any future plan to improve health services, irrespective of how radical or well-devised the plan is, *The NHS Plan* (DOH, 2000a) being no exception.

In July 2000 the Department of Health (DOH) published a document, which has been heralded as the biggest shake-up of the National Health Service (NHS) since its inception in 1948. Through its consistent and explicit emphasis throughout, on the centrality of the patient, a halt is called to the continuing conflicts that militate against this being achieved. In this radical plan for investment and reform, the DOH takes a firm stance in regard to 'old-fashioned demarcations between staff' and 'unnecessary boundaries that exist between the professions' (DOH, 2000a: 5). It asserts that these are responsible for information not being shared, investigations being repeated and delay being 'designed into the system'.

BOUNDARIES – INTRAPROFESSIONAL BARRIERS?

It seems to be the case that, in respect of boundaries, community nurses have more progress to make than others. Frequent references have been made by a number of writers over the last 20 years (Goodwin, 1983; Littlewood, 1987; King, 1990; NHS Management Executive, 1993; Newbury *et al.*, 1997) to the in-fighting and territorialism that have characterized community nursing, highlighting practitioners' involvement in *intraprofessional* conflicts and prejudices, as well as the acknowledged *interprofessional* ones.

In 1994 the United Kingdom Central Council (UKCC) claimed that, through its new educational standards and structure, it had created a 'new and unified discipline of community health care nursing' (UKCC, 1994: 13), but after a detailed scrutiny of the evidence available, Hyde (1995) argued that the claim could not be supported. She mooted the possibility that the dissimilar beliefs held firmly by some of its practitioners about community nursing, predetermined not unity, but incompatibility and conflict. After considering several reasons as to why community nurses seem to be preoccupied with differences in their identities, Hyde (1995) concluded that:

For years, community nurses have fought to establish not a collective identity, but their own unique specialist identities, thereby fostering role competition rather than role co-operation. This has engendered petty bickerings and jealousies which, in turn, have served to strengthen loyalties to membership of 'own' groups.

(Hyde, 1995: 7)

Interestingly, in its 1998 *Standards for Education and Practice* (UKCC, 1998), which renders the 1994 document 'no longer applicable' (front cover), the UKCC makes no reference to its earlier claim; but perhaps a preoccupation with the perceived strength of unity between named nurse groups is of limited relevance? The vision of *The NHS Plan* (DOH, 2000a: chapter 1) is that, rather than professionals being 'signed up' to each other (as community nurses to a 'unified discipline'), health and social services' practitioners will be 'signed up' to the client, that is, working in partnership to redesign services for the benefit of clients.

The NHS Plan

The Prime Minister set out five challenges facing the NHS; these are addressed by the ten-year *NHS Plan* (DOH, 2000a). The challenges are expressed as five 'P's, and are summarized as follows:

- *Patients*: delivering fast and convenient care for patients; listening to patients' needs and letting them know their rights.
- *Professions*: the entire NHS workforce working together to deliver services for patients; breaking down traditional barriers between healthcare professionals.
- *Performance*: taking action to set action and deliver high standards in the NHS.
- *Prevention*: promoting healthy living across all sections of society and tackling variations in care.
- *Partnership*: working together across the NHS and other services to ensure the best possible care (*National Health News*, summer 2000: 2).

The NHS Plan (DOH, 2000a) is a welcome commitment from the government to invest significant resources in the NHS. It is also a challenge to managers and practitioners to redesign the NHS structure from a model that is service-centred to one that is patient-centred. It states powerfully that: 'The frontline of healthcare is in the home' (DOH, 2000a: 2); the consequent implications for change in community nursing practice over the next ten years are vast. In order to apply the relevance of these changes to community nursing practice, in a document that gives only a token mention to a few community nursing practitioners, three themes which are threaded through *The NHS Plan* (DOH, 2000a) will be considered. The themes are:

- New ways of working.
- Public health.
- The use of health informatics to support care delivery.

NEW WAYS OF WORKING

Over the next ten years, the stated lifespan of *The NHS Plan* (DOH, 2000a), it is asserted that care delivery within patients' homes will become the norm and hospitals will become more specialized centres. The emphasis will be on promoting independence and improving the quality of care. For a national investment of £900 million, Trusts will have to demonstrate the provision of new intermediate and related care services, including:

- Intensive rehabilitation services: for example, following stroke, enabling patients to regain their health and independence.
- Recuperation facilities: within residential/nursing homes before patients return to their own homes.
- Integrated home care teams: to promote independence.
- Case management: within GP practice to ensure continuity of care.

According to Janson *et al.* (2000), the government's decision to expand intermediate care into nursing and residential homes presents a considerable challenge. These authors' research draws attention to the 'serious mismatch between the health needs of people in these homes and the services available' (p. 27). They claim that little is known about the needs, levels of service provided, or the outcomes of care for the 600 000 residents currently in nursing and residential homes, and that essentially, government surveillance of this area is missing.

This highlights a crucial role for community nurses and others involved in care management – that they work with others in the new primary care trusts (PCTs) to produce explicit guidelines and criteria that link 'reimbursement to high quality service provision' (Janson *et al.*, 2000: 26).

Integrated or fragmented care?

There is a danger that, unless primary and secondary care trusts give careful thought to the planning and implementation of an over-arching nursing strategy for their local areas, there will be a proliferation of unconnected, independent initiatives that offer care for people who live in their own homes. This would result not in the provision of seamless, integrated care, but in the fragmentation of service provision. Older people in particular, would be at risk of receiving care from separate community nursing teams and specialist nurses, none of whom is providing a comprehensive, holistic package. Already in some areas, six or more teams have been launched within short periods of time, to make specific and different contributions to the care of people in the community. For example, re-ablement teams, hospice-at-home teams and new specialist teams (e.g. for people with Parkinson's disease).

A key challenge, then, is how to enable clients to benefit from the full range of developed nursing expertise (whether acute or community-based), without compromising the continuity of care or undermining a collaborative approach. Questions must be addressed as to how the care given by different teams will be co-ordinated, and where the overall accountability lies for an individual's care. If a new team is introduced, consideration will need to be given to where it sits within the established wider healthcare team and how it might complement, and work collaboratively, with others (DOH, 1999a).

Community nurses – co-ordinators of new services?

If care is to be provided within people's homes then it could be perceived as a logical assumption by community nurses, that they will be the ones to co-ordinate it. Their qualifications as community specialist practitioners, their knowledge of the context and supporting services, and their ability to network across a complex structure of statutory and voluntary agencies, place them in a strong position. Community mental health nurses, for example, are ideally placed (given the appropriate resources) to co-ordinate and develop the 1000 graduate primary care mental health workers that *The NHS Plan* (DOH, 2000a) aims to recruit. If these 'professionally non-affiliated people' (Donnelly, 2000b: 8) are not incorporated into the existing, established structure of community mental health teams, but form an independent separate workforce, fragmentation of mental health care will be an inevitability.

Many community nurses are at the leading edge of developments in primary care and have been influential in shaping changes in nursing practice, as it responds to the wider political agenda. However, although experts in the context of care provision in the community, without considerable investment in new training and development, community nurses may lack the necessary acute nursing knowledge and skills required to develop new services. This means that monies devolved for specific projects, which require the creation of new services, such as winter planning, are created in response to political deadlines, but may not be the most appropriate way forward in the long term.

This is also evident in terminology used within *The NHS Plan* (DOH, 2000a); the term 'hospital-at- home', may indicate that the government has not quite completed its own transition in thinking from developing hospital services to truly expanding primary care teams. Secondary care trusts are developing outreach teams where patients remain the responsibility of consultants, and nursing care is provided by nurses from the acute sector with the appropriate nursing skills and knowledge; for example the Torbay Hospital Outreach Respiratory Team (THORT) has been launched by South Devon Health Care Trust for the management of patients with acute exacerbations of chronic respiratory diseases.

As a consequence of this trend, an older person presenting with multiple pathology, may, in the space of a year, receive visits from:

- A district nurse who is treating a leg ulcer.
- A respiratory team providing nursing care through an exacerbation of chronic obstructive pulmonary disease (COPD).
- A 'hospital-at-home' team administering intravenous antibiotics for cellulitis.
- A specialist nursing team which has been requested to transfuse blood.
- A community mental health nurse who is undertaking assessments relating to the onset of dementia.
- Other professionals supporting care within the home (e.g. social services, voluntary agencies).

Although a positive outcome is achieved for this person, in that an unwanted hospital admission is prevented, several negative outcomes might also result, such as disruption to the patient's routine, reduction in quality of life or confusion due to too many strangers.

A review of district nursing services in England and Wales (Audit Commission, 1999: 98) considers various schemes and highlights the fact that if district nursing is to be able to respond to increasing and changing care provision within the home there needs to be a shift in 'whole system' budgets, to primary care. Dialogue between primary care groups (PCGs) or PCTs and secondary care providers, is going to be an essential key; this will prevent the development of independent teams, whose sole focus is their individual expertise. If success is to be attained in the pursuit of a patient-centred model then patients must have a named professional who is responsible for all aspects of their care co-ordination and delivery, and for the provision of advice and support. Opportunities for joint working need to be embraced, in order to ensure a better understanding of patients' needs and the provision of high-quality continuous care. This has implications.

Expanding roles

The NHS Plan (DOH, 2000a: chapters 7 and 9) issues a clear challenge to previous cultures and ways of working, in particular the hierarchical structure that has existed between doctors and nurses. It demands 'radical changes . . . in the way that staff work' and requires 'a commitment of individuals not just organisations'. It behoves individual community nurses then, to consider the opportunities that the Chief Nursing Officer's ten key roles offer, to both develop their expertise and clinical-decision making skills, and reflect critically on embedded culture and practice. The ten roles are:

1. To order diagnostic investigations such as pathology tests and X-rays
2. To make and receive referrals direct, e.g. a therapist, pain consultant.
3. To admit and discharge patients for specified conditions using protocols.
4. To manage patient caseloads, e.g. diabetes, rheumatology.
5. To run clinics, e.g. ophthalmology, dermatology
6. To prescribe medicines and treatments.
7. To carry out a wide range of resuscitation procedures.
8. To perform minor surgery and outpatient procedures.
9. To triage patients using the latest information technology (IT) to the most appropriate professional.
10. To take a lead in the way the local health services are organized and in the way that they are run.

The NHS Plan (DOH, 2000a) states that 'pressure on GP services will be eased as nurses and other community staff . . . take on more tasks'. This implies an unquestioning, automatic acceptance on the part of community nurses, but a cautious stance should be adopted. If the driving force is nothing more than the need to free up doctors' time, and the outcome is not the provision of a more holistic *nursing* service to patients then these additional tasks and related roles should be resisted strongly. The 'tasks' must remain integral to the provision of nursing care and not become isolated as a convenient delegation of GPs' responsibilities. The expansion of roles for community nurses must bring clinical decision-making closer to patients. It is easy to deduce that empowering community nurses to refer, admit and discharge, and order diagnostics will reduce delays in the system and that, alongside the ability to prescribe, either independently as with district nurses and health visitors, or under group protocols will enable patients to receive timely treatment.

Collaborative working

The NHS Plan (DOH, 2000a) clearly demonstrates the government's commitment to the provision of a seamless service and bridging the *barriers* that have existed in the last ten years since the implementation of the Community Care Act (DOH, 1990). The vision of a 24-hour, seven days a week, 365 days a year, integrated health and social service, designed around the needs of the patient is supported throughout. The requirement for professionals to integrate care assessments and care plans will provide a foundation for collaborative working.

The *barriers* that need to be bridged are the divisions between the NHS and social care, that is, *interorganizational*, and those within the NHS, that is, *intraorganizational*. According to the Audit Commission (2000) report on rehabilitation and remedial services for older people the need for better joint planning between health and social services has long been recognized. However, what is less well-recognized is that many of the difficulties occur because of discontinuities between different parts of the NHS. The *barriers* between acute and community health services, and between acute and primary care services, can be every bit as high as those between health and social care.

Walsh *et al.* (2000), the national personal medical services evaluation study team, found this to be the case in regard to the first 14 personal medical services pilot schemes that had been 'slow to develop links with key organisations' (Walsh *et al.*, 2000: 28). These authors noted 'limited evidence of closer relationships between PMS provider organisations and other services within the NHS'. Yet again, *barriers* were encountered and joint working had been obstructed by 'internally focused' people with vested interests.

Despite the repeated reference to *barriers*, there are several examples that indicate that those who perpetuate them are not necessarily representative of the wider professions. These examples are exciting and signify that many are casting aside boundaries and territories, having realized that divisions divide and exclude colleagues, and collaboration achieves the opposite:

Example 1
In Fife, area and staff boundaries were crossed (Davies, 1998), when a multiprofessional group from hospitals, the community and nursing homes established a wound care forum which is now attended by approximately

60 people; it is open to all disciplines and attendees come from a range of backgrounds.

Example 2
Phillips and Frith (2000) report on a multiprofessional management development programme in the Trent region, which is evaluated as a positive experience for doctors (second- and third-year specialist registrars and GP trainees), managers, finance specialists, nurses and professions allied to medicine. They found that 'with time and willingness on the part of individuals, attitudes were found to change' (p. 23). These are just two of hundreds of refreshing collaborative initiatives that would seem to indicate the readiness of increasing numbers of workers, to embrace new ways of working.

Integrated care pathways

The importance of how community nurses work with the multidisciplinary team has been established. However, new ways of thinking are also required in regard to:

- Predictability of specific care requirements, e.g. following stroke, myocardial infarction.
- Reasonable timescales in which certain outcomes can be expected.
- Evidence-based practice incorporating locally agreed standards.
- Quality assurance.
- Supporting documentation.

Various definitions of integrated care pathways (Johnson, 1997; Currie and Harvey, 1998; Middleton and Roberts, 1998), include the above aspects of care provision and provide a fresh approach to the way in which care is delivered. Community nurses must consider their contribution to the development of care pathways and the consequent benefits and constraints of this way of working. Browning and Hollingbury (2000: 34) exemplify the way in which integrated care pathways provide the opportunity to examine care processes and outcomes, and clarify standards of care. The potential benefits which Browning and Hollingbury (2000) identify, such as setting out what clinicians do, seeing if we all do the same thing, agreeing with the same things, challenging what we do, and comparing it to the evidence base, could be seen by others as a threat to individual autonomy (Jones, 1999). Jones (1999) continues to argue that particularly within mental health services the predictability of conditions is not always certain enough to render integrated care pathways viable. National service frameworks, such as that for coronary heart disease (DOH, 2000b), lend themselves to providing the basis for integrated care pathways to be developed. It is important that community nurses grasp the significance of each national service framework in their everyday working practices and are able to contribute to the development of integrated care pathways. Care pathways are also a means by which poor resources can be identified in a constructive way (Currie and Harvey, 1998) and may give community nurses the opportunity to have an impact on standards of care.

NHS Direct

Significantly, the role of NHS Direct (a nurse-led advisory telephone service (DOH, 1997)) is to be further developed as 'a one-stop gateway to health-care' (DOH, 1997: 2). This is of concern to GPs who rightly perceive that it will have a direct effect on their workload and professional judgement (Greenwood, 2000). The plan also suggests that NHS Direct will be developed from an advice line prompted by an individual's call to a more proactive source of nursing support, particularly to the elderly, 'NHS Direct nurses will be in regular contact . . . and check that older people living alone are all right.' (DOH, 1997: 2). Community nurses should share the same concerns as GPs and consider their own accountability framework. The roles of NHS Direct nurses in the future, will have significant overlap with the roles of community nurses (e.g. to help patients manage their medicines and advise on care at home), and for this reason the relationship between NHS Direct nurses and community nurses must be made explicit. McKenna (2000) encourages clinicians to see the potential for NHS Direct to contribute to existing services, and challenges them to work with and help shape its development. Given that McKenna (2000) asserts that NHS Direct will have a profound effect on how the NHS will evolve, it is imperative that community nurses take up this challenge.

Making a Difference (DOH, 1999), a strategy for nurses, midwives and health visitors, does not offer any specific direction for NHS Direct nurses in terms of context, training requirements, skills or experience. It also neglects to comment on the impact that recruitment to NHS Direct (a brand new nursing career pathway) will have on the retention of nurses in other areas.

PUBLIC HEALTH

In Chapter 2, Mason has offered a working definition of public health for nurses as: 'organized social and political effort, and health promotion for the benefit of populations, families and individuals'. She concludes that community nursing incorporates aspects of public health work but is primarily client- and family-centred rather than population-centred. In *The NHS Plan* (DOH, 2000a) community nurses are required to examine the scope to adopt a public health approach in their practice.

The public health nursing title is attributed to health visitors by the UKCC (1998), but increasingly, is recognized as part of the role of school nurses (DOH, 1999b). However, other community nurses should be encouraged to focus on the wider determinants of health, to consider how they affect their particular client groups and to widen their networks to incorporate other relevant agencies such as housing and environmental health. *The NHS Plan* (DOH, 2000a) promises a new leadership programme that will provide community nurses with 'the skills and expertise to work directly with representatives of local neighbourhood and housing estates to support communities and improve health'. However, local health improvement teams and multi-agency partnerships (including local authorities, social services or the police, for example), whose purpose is to consider priorities such as coronary heart disease, cancer, promoting independence, preventing accidents, childrens' services (Teignbridge Primary Care Group, 1999) are examples of how community nurses are already contributing to the public health agenda.

Community nurses are being challenged to examine their roles and explore new ways of working. However it may not be their own lack of creativity that disables them from contributing to the public health agenda. District nurses, for example, may be perceived by others as solely providing a clinical service, the development of a public health role being a diversion from their core skills (Caraher and Allen, 2000). Time constraints may therefore impinge on any public health activity and staffing resources, preventing any dedicated public health research or work. Morgan and Rowe (1998) encourage members of primary health care teams that they could be:

A powerful force for addressing the health needs of groups and communities, for considering the structural causes of health and for considering an individual's health in the context of the broad nature of health and well being.

(Morgan and Rowe, 1998: 28)

The way in which community nurses are required to record work activity, that is, by patient contact, may also prevent time being spent on other activities such as public health work. Methods of recording this aspect of their role must be developed and valued as integral to the appropriate development of community nursing services of the future.

Access to healthcare will be 'measured and managed' by 2001 (DOH, 2000a) and community nurses must appraise how their services are accessed. For example, is it appropriate to be a 'referred-to' service? This may be felt to be a way of rationing care provision in areas where teams are already working beyond their capacity. However, if community nurses cultivate a public health approach to their work and are allocated the time and resources to reach people that would otherwise have fallen through the net the potential for reducing inequalities can be exploited.

THE USE OF HEALTH INFORMATICS TO SUPPORT CARE DELIVERY

The purpose of a robust information strategy for the NHS is clearly defined by the NHS strategy, *Information for Health* (NHSE, 1998). This provides the framework for developments in health informatics, streamlining the exchange of professional communication and information via an individualized electronic patient record that will enable the delivery of seamless care to patients. In time it will also support the development of health improvement programmes (HImPs) that underpin the work of the NHS (DOH, 1997), by providing data which has been 'aggregated and placed into anonymised subsets' (DOH, 1998: 4) for public health data collection and analysis. The government has committed £200 million to modernizing IT systems (DOH,

2000a) and, by 2004, it is anticipated that 75% of secondary care trusts and 50% of primary care and community care services will have implemented the electronic patient record. There are two issues that need to be addressed for community nurses:

- Can nurse leaders articulate the kind of information required that will be meaningful to community nurses and other professionals providing care?
- Do all nurses have the relevant computing skills that will enable them to input data efficiently?

Alpay *et al.* (2000) provide a timely review of issues and trends in the use of IT by nurses working in primary care and encourage community nurses to become proactive in its development. It is essential, these authors claim, that community nurses grasp the implications of the electronic patient record and ensure that the programmes are developed in a way that enables them to best describe the care that they deliver, and that they can derive from it the information that is pertinent to enhancing the care community nurses provide. The review by Alpay *et al.* (2000) highlights key issues that urgently need to be addressed: community nurses' attitudes towards IT; changes in working practices, and the education and training needs of community nurses. It is vital that community nurses are empowered to understand the broader potential of IT and how it might enhance multiprofessional working (Saranto, 1998). The vision of *The NHS Plan* (DOH, 2000a) is that the electronic patient records will 'enable nurses, therapists and doctors to maintain continuity of care and knowledge of their patients' (p. 2). Community nurses must grasp the opportunity to lead in the development of the primary care programmes, otherwise they may find themselves repeating negative experiences, such as multiple data collection programmes that cannot be accessed; GP programmes which are not designed for community nurse input or inputting data on multiple systems concurrently in order to satisfy different information and communication needs.

Addressing the education and training needs of community nurses with regard to IT must be seen as fundamental to continuing professional development and not as an aside that is undertaken only if there is time. If the Chief Nursing Officer's ten key roles for nurses are to be developed and taken seriously by others, nurses must be able to use the latest IT that supports care delivery. It could be seen as an oversight that although *Making a Difference* (DOH, 1999) acknowledges that there is an 'information revolution' (p. 8) there is no specific reference in the chapter (pp 23–31) to strengthening education and training in IT. *The NHS Plan* (DOH, 2000a) finally recognizes that clinical staff need the 'time and space to redesign and reorganise their services'; this must include supporting staff to use IT systems that support patient care. Despite the negative attitudes of community nurses towards IT identified by Alpay *et al.* (2000), a huge commitment is needed from managers and community nurses alike to add IT training into core individual development plans.

The focus of this last section has been on IT and it would be easy to lose a sense that care is being redesigned around patients. However, effective communication systems between professionals, that support seamless care delivery, are fundamental whether by personal, paper or electronic methods. Community nurses must remain proactive in the IT agenda to ensure that advances in IT are appropriate to patients' needs and remain as a support to service development and not a means to an end.

Conclusion

It seems that the biggest challenge to ensuring the success of The NHS Plan (DOH, 2000a), and the modernization of the NHS to be a responsive, patient-centred service, is the breaking down of barriers. Without real and continued commitment to collaborative working, none of the five challenges (patients, professionals, performance, prevention and partnership) addressed by The NHS Plan (DOH, 2000a), can be fully met. As stated at the beginning of the chapter, the potential for the development of community nursing is unprecedented.

In the words of Fatchett (1996: 41), community nurses are faced with two choices: 'to do nothing and let others determine their future as a profession', or to 'create a strategy that puts them in . . . control of their roles'. If they choose the latter, their influence on both the shape of community nursing in the new NHS and the success of The NHS Plan (DOH, 2000a) will be substantial.

References

Alpay, L., Needham, G. and Murray, P. (2000) Information technology for nurses in primary care. Primary Health Care Research and Development, 1: 5–13.

Audit Commission. (1999) First assessment – a review of district nursing services in England and Wales. London: Audit Commission.

Audit Commission. (2000) The way to go home: rehabilitation and remedial services for older people. London: The Stationery Office.

Browning, R. and Hollingbury, T. (2000) For good measure. Health Service Journal, 110: 34–5.

Caraher, M. and Allen, D. (2000) District nurses and the new public health agenda. Primary Nursing Care, January: 18–21.

Castledine, G. (1999) A nursing 'peace' vs the medical 'war' model. British Journal of Nursing, 8: 62.

Castledine, G. (2000) PAMs are concerned about nurse consultants. British Journal of Nursing, 9: 382.

Cumberlege, J. (1990) Collaboration. London: Centre for the Advancement of Interprofessional Education (CAIPE).

Currie, L. and Harvey, G. (1998) Care pathway development and implementation. Nursing Standard, 12: 15–21.

Dalley, G. (1993) Professional ideology or organisational tribalism? The health service –social work divide. In: Walmsley, J., Reynolds, J., Shakespeare, P. and Woolfe, R. (eds) Health, welfare and practice. Buckingham: Open University/Sage.

Davies, D. (1998) Crossing area and staff boundaries in wound care. *Professional Nurse*, 13: 472–3.

Department of Health (DOH). (1990) *NHS and community care act*. London: HMSO.

Department of Health (DOH). (1997) *The new NHS – modern and dependable*. London: The Stationery Office.

Department of Health (DOH). (1999a) *Making a difference – strengthening the nursing, midwifery and health visiting contribution to health and healthcare*. London: The Stationery Office.

Department of Health (DOH). (1999b) *Saving lives: our healthier nation*. London: DOH.

Department of Health (DOH). (2000a) *The NHS Plan*. London: The Stationery Office.

Department of Health (DOH). (2000b) *National service frameworks: coronary heart disease*. London: DOH.

Dixon, C. (1998) Time for some lateral thinking. *Community Practitioner*, 71: 282.

Donnelly, L. (2000a) Talking it through. *Health Service Journal*, 110: 11–12.

Donnelly, L. (2000b) 'Extra resources needed' to meet future demands on mental health. *Health Service Journal*, 110: 8–9.

Eaton, L. (1999) Working together. *Community Practitioner*, 72: 7–8.

Fatchett, A. (1996) A chance for community nurses to shape the health agenda. *Nursing Times*, 92: 40–2.

Frith, K. and Frith, J. (2000) Changes attitudes takes time and willingness. *Health Service Journal*, 110: 23.

Goodwin, S. (1983) Away with the velvet jacket brigade. *Nursing Mirror*, 156: 26.

Greenwood, L. (2000) IT looks like trouble. *Health Service Journal*, 110: 13–14.

Howkins, E. (1995) Collaborative care: an agreed goal, but a difficult journey. In: Cain, P., Hyde, V. and Howkins, E. (eds) *Community nursing: dimensions and dilemmas*. London: Arnold.

Hyde, V. (1995) Community nursing: a unified discipline? In: Cain, P., Hyde, V. and Howkins, E. (eds) *Community nursing: dimensions and dilemmas*. London: Arnold.

Janson, K., Law, Watts, C. and Pollock, A. (2000) Lost and confused. *Health Service Journal*, 110: 26–9.

Johnson, S. (1997) *Pathways of care*. Oxford: Blackwell Science.

Jones, A. (1999) The development of mental health care pathways – friend or foe? *British Journal of Nursing*, 8: 1441–3.

King, D. (1990) Teamwork in primary care. *Nursing*, 4: 36–7.

Littlewood, J. (1987) Community nursing – an overview. In: Littlewood, J. (ed.) *Recent advances in nursing: community nursing*. Edinburgh: Churchill Livingstone; 1–26.

Lockhart-Wood, K. (2000) Collaboration between nurses and doctors in clinical practice. *British Journal of Nursing*, 9: 276–80.

McDonald, A., Langford, I. and Boldero, N. (1997) The future of community nursing in the United Kingdom. *Journal of Advanced Nursing*, 26: 257–65.

McKenna, K. (2000) Calling clinicians to help shape NHS Direct – and overcome your concerns. *Health Service Journal*, 110: 23.

Middleton, S. and Roberts, A. (1998) *Clinical pathways workbook*. Clinical Pathways Reference Centre.

Morgan, M. and Rowe, A. (1998) Is public health work possible within primary health care teams? In: CPHVA *Poverty and public health; finally on the agenda*. London: CPHVA; 25–8.

Newbury, J., Clarridge, A. and Skinner, J. (1997) Collaboration for care. In Burley, S., Mitchell, E.E., Melling, K., Smith, M., Chilton, S. and Crumplin, C. (eds.) *Contemporary community nursing*. London: Arnold.

NHS Management Executive (1993) *New world, new opportunities: nursing in primary health care*. London: HMSO.

NHS Executive (1998) *Information for health – an information strategy for the modern NHS*. London: NHSE.

Parkin, P. (1999) Managing change in the community 1: the case of PCGs. *British Journal of Community Nursing*, 4: 19–27.

Saranto, K. (1998) Outcomes of education in information technology at nursing polytechnics. *Health Informatics Journal*, 4: 84–91.

Teignbridge Primary Care Group. (2000) Teignbridge health improvement programme. In: South and West Devon Health Authority. *Better health and well being*. Dartington: SAWDHA.

United Kingdom Central Council (UKCC). (1994) *The future of professional practice – the Council's standards for education and practice following registration*. London: UKCC.

United Kingdom Central Council (UKCC). (1998) *Standards for specialist education and practice*. London: UKCC.

Walsh, N., Huntington, J., Barnes, M., Baines, D. and Rogers, H. (2000) Friends and relations. *Health Service Journal*, 110: 28–9.

Index

Note: abbreviations used in the index are: CPA = care programme approach; GPs = general practitioners; HImPs = health improvement programmes; PCGs = primary care groups; PCTs = primary care trusts.